SHUT UP & OBEY

DIGGING DEEPER INTO THE CONTROVERSIAL LOCKDOWN

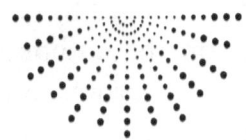

SKYE ANGELOU

CONTENTS

Introduction   ix

1. The History of Vaccine Injuries   1
2. Digging Deep into the Controversial
   Lockdown   14
3. Finding a Balance – Restricting the
   People's Liberties   33
4. The Impact Of The Controversial
   Lockdown On Covid-19 Spread   39
5. Limited Trust - Vaccines Big Pharma
   Cooperation   65
6. Vaccine Liberty—The People's
   Choice   73
7. Covid-19 Politics – Who Called The
   Shots?   78
8. Pursuing a Natural Solution   95
9. Reflecting on the Pandemic   101
10. Where Do We Go From Here?   111
11. Conclusion   130
12. About the Author   134

INTRODUCTION

There is no absolute guarantee of anything man made, not even medical intervention will when solving a problem. In fact, the risk associated with medical intervention is higher, and vaccines are no different. Vaccines can cause serious to minor to non-existent side effects such as swelling, allergy, and itching at the injection site, and some have shown life-threatening reactions, even death.

When vaccines were introduced to humans as a cure option, there was almost no compensation for vaccine injuries as it was still in its infancy. This gave room for gross negligence and disregard until the 1902 US Biologics Control Act came into the picture. Even with its policy, vaccine injuries persist, and lawsuits are not unheard of.

Healing is nature's gift to everyone—to you, to me, to all of us—but our negligence is a marketing point for the big Pharma companies. We will fall sick, but we are ill because we ignore the signs our body emits. Like so many things in human life, we do not give a hoot until it is beyond our control. Sometimes it feels like we love it when we are suddenly dependent and love to tell stories of overcoming a tragedy or condition.

In my previous book, The Untold Secrets to Healing, I narrate a story about a loved one who suffered so much pain until my aunt defied the doctor's reports and sought to heal herself, and in no time, my cousin was jumping around, and doctors termed it a "miracle." It amazes me why they never think of or want to acknowledge other medicinal or healing sources.

Sometimes we learn through suffering and discomfort, but we cannot sweep the matter of vaccine injuries under the rug anymore. It has been a long time coming, but the pandemic was the straw that broke the camel's back.

We are surrounded by a cloak of lies, fake information, and farce that the world or a group of people want to see. Regardless of their motives for pushing a lie, it is time to open their eyes to the truth.

And What Are Those Truths?

I beg for your indulgence and open-mindedness when reading this book. This is not an opportunity to propagate another or extend the conspiracy theories flying in the air, but for people to look closely and question the mechanics of the systems around them. We are, unfortunately, trapped in a system that will do anything to prevent you and me from learning about the truth. This process has been a long time coming, as policies, laws, systems, and punishments are in place to quiet anyone that dares to say otherwise. But we are speaking up! And yes, they call them conspiracy theories. However, there is an element of truth in every rumor.

The pandemic vaccine is the biggest vaccine hoax ever. I have seen people fall sicker after each flu shot. A friend had the vaccine and was sick with the flu. She got tested, and the result said she had COVID. She took another shot, got sick again, and was told to take another Covid shot.

Unbelievable! When did we get here? And yet, many of you do not see that the vaccine is damaging us—making us sicker and sicker.

People, we are not free—we live under the illusion of freedom. We live in a small prison, like rats in a test lab, where we think we are free because we move around as we want but are thoroughly limited by what we can access, own, or acquire. Even though it feels like we have freedom, there are masters behind the scenes, like puppeteers pulling the strings. We extended the strings to them, unbeknownst to many of us, and sank deeper and deeper into enslavement.

There was a time when the masters needed the masses to work and produce, but technology has made us obsolete; now we have become, in Mr. Harari's own words, "useless people," and according to them, there are far too many of us.

THE HISTORY OF VACCINE INJURIES

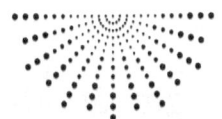

2020, 2021, and 2022 were confusing years for many; employees were frazzled by the government's insistence on a vaccine, and employers had fewer workers as many refused the vaccine.

We were in the middle of the biggest conspiracy, fraud, and cover-up ever, and as we tried to make sense, the government brought forth policies that hampered us and kept us locked down. You could work with a COVID VAX, which meant no income and the ability to cater for yourself or your family. It was a choice to do as they wanted despite the ever-increasing rates of vaccine injuries, disabilities, and death among the vaccinated.

In history, there was a mass genocide taking place under the guise of mass vaccination. A larger part of the population did not know what was happening and was coerced into wearing a mask, taking a jab, and being tested. Most people who lost their loved ones in the hospital under the guise of the COVID virus never got to see or even have an autopsy conducted on their bodies.

The pandemic brought another bout of global immunization. Now do not get it twisted, immunization has saved the lives of millions throughout the ages and in curbing the reoccurrence of the disease. Many have lived because of them, but the Covid-19 vaccine is different. We do not have access to Covid information, how it works, how it is made, how long it remains effective, and the side effects. Furthermore, doctors and medical committees, and associations are even more in the dark than the citizens.

Either way, someone is lying and it is not us – we are on the receiving end. There is a huge agenda and skepticism about the government and global elite to manage the world's population. We are not ignorant that science is capable of creating and recreating even diseases and we are the test subjects.

The WHO (World Health Organization) was so confused, it kept coming up with excuses; lockdown, no lockdown, putting everyone at risk. Such incompetence from the people we have easily handed our lives to cannot be tolerated.

Even when people died from the effect of the Vaccine, the government turned a blind eye. They took our loved ones and prevented us from seeing them. We only heard they did not make it.

They buried our dead. They misinformed us. They lied and are still lying about COVID and the vaccine. Perhaps one of the most surprising pieces of information was that we had to force our kids to get vaccinated with parental consent. WHY?

Why would any sane government go to such a hideous length just to vaccinate its population secretly? They know that to carry out their World Agenda program, they need children to rebel against their parents by brainwashing them into believing that they have their rights and are independent under the law.

The CDC has been lying to the population for years, and the COVID vaccine is no different. According to a global research statement, the US

CDC did not count victims that died after the first jab if they passed 14 days before the second Pfizer or Modena shot. The truth is that many cases of vaccine injuries and deaths happen within this time window. While this is a lie, it inflates the death rate of unvaccinated individuals and hides the real danger of the COVID vaccines.

I have many stories from people who suffered severely from the COVID vaccine. My problem is that nobody sees the wrong that the government is doing to the people. How do they want to enforce protection against the people's will? I guess even democracy has some lapses.

So I read this story about a guy who said that five of his loved ones got sick or died from the vaccine, and the funny side of this story was that he was with every one of them (all infected with COVID) and did not get the virus or gets vaccinated. His friend died after his doctor pressed him, another died from high blood pressure, and his father-in-law had a severe heart attack, yet we say the government is transparent.

We need to wake up!

Guillain-Barré syndrome struck a vibrant woman and grandmother. It was pathetic seeing her behave like an imbecile and not even be able to feed herself. There are many more stories like these, yet nobody—not the government, big Pharma companies, or health regulatory bodies—is saying anything about them.

We are just pawns in their hands to push an agenda of global depopulation and a new world order. I am not asking you to believe it but just think for a moment.

Vaccines have helped many of us survive debilitating illnesses such as polio, chicken pox, smallpox, and even the flu, but with the COVID vaccine, the story is different, some gaps cannot be explained.

Despite our awareness of the dangers of vaccines throughout history, people still went ahead to get the vaccine without the proper information. Until recently, the injuries caused by the vaccine were kept under wraps, but many people suffered from TTS (thrombosis with thrombocytopenia syndrome), which is blood clotting in various organs. Another injury triggered by the vaccine jab is the Guillain-Barré syndrome, where the immune system attacks the peripheral nervous system.

Myocarditis is a common complaint among people who received the mRNA COVID vaccine. This is a condition in which the heart becomes inflamed within days of receiving the vaccine, primarily in younger male adults. In each injury case, the side effects were noticeable a few days or weeks after receiving the jab. Some are still wondering if this is true, but for those who have loved ones that suffered from the vaccine's adverse effects; their thought is what will happen to people later, in the coming months or years.

Even after everything, many job candidates refused to get jobs because a major factor in being employed was taking the vaccine.

Where are our freedom and right of choice?

If the vaccine was "good," why enforce it? I cannot wrap my head around how people still fall for this lie the government is telling us. Anyway, I refuse to judge anyone, but this is literally what happens when we trust the government and policymakers more than God or what nature has offered. It is past time for us to take a step back and reflect deeply on the doctrine that society is selling to us.

If you don't believe in Covid vaccines, why are there so many Covid vaccine injury compensation claims everywhere—from the United States to Canada to the United Kingdom—and why are vaccine documents difficult to find online?

Like many other sectors of our lives, the health authorities and government are trying to normalize the sudden deaths of vaccinated people, especially young people. These are young people who were healthy and doing well until they were forced to get the jab, avoid work, or access public places.

The vaccines were proclaimed safe, but how safe are they? The FDA and big Pharma companies asked for 75 years to produce public documents on COVID and vaccines. My take is that there is something wrong, and they need time to polish up dirty surfaces and tie up loose ends. We have such sophisticated computing systems, yet they need almost a century to gather information for public consumption.

Wondering why?

Furthermore, the vaccine makers are indemnified by the government. Despite the injury claims received and paid to victims, people still do not believe in the truth that the COVID-19 vaccine is a hoax and a sham perpetrated by the government as an agenda for a sinister purpose.

Rather than incite an uprising against the government as some manipulators would say, the purpose of this book is to reveal the hidden truth about the Covid-19 pandemic and enlighten you about government propaganda regarding the vaccine.

One major tool that has been used to rope people into taking vaccines against their will is misinformation. Being confined to our homes as safety measures to prevent the transmission of the virus, we are unable to fact-check whatever we see on TV and it has given the government and media agencies ample space to pervert the truth that Covid-19 might not be as deadly as they pointed out or might just be a cover-up for something more insidious. It is no secret that the world's population is slowly approaching an optimal position, but is mass genocide approved as a means of population control? These conversations must be brought to light.

If the virus was truly easily spread through human contact, areas with dense populations and less advanced societies would have experienced a higher death rate. According to predictions, African countries were meant to experience alarming death rates but their numbers were millions below Europe and Asia. This creates many questions for westerners to answer. Are Africans immune to the disease? Is there a different variation per continent? Was the disease just a scam that African leaders refused to sign up for? How exactly did Africa get through the pandemic without recording even a quarter of the losses in other continents? The answer to this would be that Covid-19 is fake or there is a cure in Africa that is hidden from the world at large.

Over tens of millions of deaths have been reported from Covid-19 infections, but what the media houses don't report too is that almost a quarter of that number died after taking the jab. Why would a vaccine that is meant to cure or protect one against a disease, be the cause of death in the end? Some things are unclear. The numbers of recorded deaths rank around 17 million people upwards, but this is not the worst that the world has handled. Coming from centuries when Polio, Flu, HIV, and the Black Death ravaged the world, we are dealing with much less and there are still so many knowledge gaps unlike in the past century.

The deadliest of these happens to be the Black Death which claimed about 50 million lives at a time when the world population was lesser than it is. The plague traveled on the wings of infected fleas and flew across borders much in the same way that Covid was taken on planes, and the death of victims seemed impossible to stop, but in the end, and after two other reoccurrences, vaccines were created.

However, the vaccines were not given for public use but rather to health workers and people who risked exposure to infected animals or ports. If a deadlier disease was managed successfully like that, then we must see that the government is force-feeding everyone the vaccine for reasons unknown.

Some theories carried on the internet are that Corona Virus indeed is real but wasn't as deadly and resistant to diseases in the beginning until the government began to privately mutate these strains to create deadlier and more resistant variants. The result of this was that even the people who had taken the vaccine were more susceptible to the newer strains than those who had not taken the jab yet.

In other words, the vaccine was a preparation field for the strains to come and made the people easier targets. This is asides from the already noted side effects which range from hemorrhages, fever, and the possibility of Covid-19 amongst other nervous and respiratory problems.

Another rumor about the origins of the virus is that it was the result of a government effort to create a bioweapon that went out of hand and is being covered up under the guise of a pandemic. Regardless of this, fewer reports rose about the vaccine's effectiveness in late 2020 and early 2021 and the government still mandated it notwithstanding the negative side effects.

The possible reasons why this instruction prevailed asides from depopulation include Economic gains. At the crux of the pandemic and the global lockdown, the more buoyant governments distributed funds to their citizens but prioritized the vaccinated people first. Similarly lesser developed countries obliged with the distribution of the vaccines even though they had relatively low cases of the virus because they wanted to benefit from the relief materials and funds from elite individuals, world banks, and health organizations like the WHO.

The government and big pharma guns turned a blind eye to the number of people who reported that they still got infected after taking the vaccines or died from the jabs. It quickly became a requirement for international travel and since the UK, USA, and Canada were championing the movement, none of the smaller countries wanted to be on their bad books. What was at play wasn't that the governments cared anymore about health or the pandemic, but instead they focused on strengthening bonds, receiving relief money, and ensuring that the Covid-19 agenda prospered.

In most cases, the disease could be combated with strong supplements and antibiotics at the initial stages of contact, so what was the need for a vaccine with negative effects and possible death? I have asked this question repeatedly and the answer is that the governments were covering something up.

It could be that the virus and vaccine were already subtly being used as bio-weapons and deployed to specific areas that they wanted to wipe out like beta testing. Perhaps the religious fanatics had a point when they screamed about a sort of satanic initiation spoken of in the Bible, although that is pretty far-fetched. The point is that they realized very quickly that something else was at play. Nobody was denied job opportunities because they didn't have a vaccine for the bubonic plague or others. The disease was very deadly and people willingly opted for the vaccine which was properly tested and safe to use. But it seems more like the Covid Vaccine is a dangerous ticket to death and sickness that people reject.

I am not in on the COVID vaccine, as I believe there is more to it than meets the eye. It is not about mainstream media or what was said or not said in the media, but the inability of the government to open up about the virus despite living in a modern and innovative world. This book is designed to be read carefully and absorbed into your system, but it is also meant to help you ask questions and learn more about our environment.

We will thrive when we understand that we are slaves and accept anything that is said without questioning the process and protocols.

2
DIGGING DEEP INTO THE CONTROVERSIAL LOCKDOWN

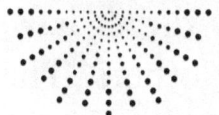

*T*he COVID lockdown was a prudent precautionary measure by the government to mitigate the spread of the virus, but it was also the riskiest test ever conducted on the public in a long time. Despite researchers' warnings that the lockdown would prove deadlier then the pandemic, they still went ahead with it. Aside from the increase in unemployment and businesses, cases of domestic abuse went up, and many people died of diseases like heart conditions, pneumonia, and cancer because they could not afford doctors and medication to treat them.

But the sad truth is that scientists and the government were willing to take such a risk without weighing the dangers. There have been no significant benefits to date, indicating that the lockdown was successful. Early in the pandemic, WHO recommended that face masks are worn by health workers or people confirmed with the virus to stop the spread, but later changed its opinion and made it mandatory for everyone to contain the spread.

There were many psychological impacts from the lockdown, and I can tell you that they were all negative. Nobody enjoyed the lockdown except for lazy people or people with outdoor phobias.

One of the most heinous consequences of the lockdown was the fear of contracting the disease and the number of people who were victim to the virus. Fear was the reason many people were hospitalized for symptoms that were not COVID under the guise of the virus, and many died in fear. If the lockdown did anything good, kids had lots of playtimes as schools and educational facilities were also locked down.

However, there were limitations on freedom based on implicit orders by the government and health directors that resulted in relationship deterioration as we could not approach our loved ones, hug them, eat together, or place our aging parents in care homes. Human beings are social animals, and we thrive by socializing and interacting with one another; this was one aspect that questioned the virus. Why would any sickness keep you away from your loved one?

While many people say or think the government did the right thing, we still had deaths that ran into the hundreds of thousands. There were countries like Sweden that refused to implement the lockdown and yet had the lowest COVID death rate.

Why was it?

When the pandemic shut down the world and lockdown laws were imposed across the country, Sweden went in the opposite direction, continuing to live as usual years after the so-called Sweden experiment. They suffered the consequences but also handled it better than many countries.

Some aspects of the lockdown that weren't right are:

- Putting on the face masks

Lets have a closer look at the masks:

The virus spreads by droplets transmitted in the air through coughs, sneezes, or speaking, and to curb this spread, face masks were made mandatory in the US and many other countries around the world. There has been so much debate on the effectiveness of masks to curb the virus that certain peer reviews validate the use of masks for protection.

In fact, a study showed that while the mask prevented the virus from being spread, it did not stop the wearer from inhaling the virus and getting COVID. Additionally, wearing a mask gave a false sense of security, making people ignore many other aspects necessary for controlling the infection.

On the flip side, wearing a mask hinders breathing flow as exhaled air goes into the eyes, which generates the impulse to want to scratch your eyes or rub them (a no-no for the pandemic region) because your hands could be contaminated. It also goes against the World Health Organization's mask warnings and measures. Also, wearing a mask meant deeper breathing, which is good without the pandemic but is risky as infected people could spread the virus deeper than normal.

- Immunity

Though the lockdown was to safeguard us, it also kept us away from activities that could help us heal and fight the virus. The controversial lockdown meant we could not naturally increase the power of our immune system. Several studies discovered that neutralizing antibodies remained high after infection but would gradually drop as time passed. However, a peer review out of China showed that infected people suffered steep declines in antibody levels within 8 to 12 weeks of infection. This meant the vaccine could not provide lasting immunity as repeated doses were needed to wash off the virus.

I have to speak about the "Got Milk" ads again. Remember how celebrities promoted the benefits of milk including its essence for bone health? Later, they said milk is not good for us and our bones.

That certainly left many of us mouth agape but my point is the same celebrities are promoting the jab. Wonder what they will say 5 or 10 years down the line when they realize it was all the manipulation of global elite and government agencies?

The government agenda was to impose the vaccine on everyone by force based on boosting the immune system, and allowing people to go about their activities would make that agenda useless, so the lockdown was imposed.

Let's take a look:

The lockdown kept us inside to avoid the spread of the disease, which was supposedly crucial.

Lack of connection to nature and Vitamin D

The pandemic required that we remain indoors and away from natural light, air, and nature. As a simple way of combating diseases, this meant fewer social interactions. While these effects were good, they missed an integral aspect of human wellness. Many people suffer from a weakened immune system and increased stress due to a lack of vitamin D. We must understand that the body functions like a clock, with night and day phases. By staying indoors, we are automatically altering the body's ability to produce Vitamin D, a vital component for healthy bones, teeth, immune cells, and our defense against infection.

A bunch of scientists, experts in their respective fields, took the initiative to lock us in because maybe, just maybe, we could defeat this virus on our own. They shut down our body's mechanisms, making us susceptible to infections, especially respiratory-related ones. Once you got into the hospital for the flu or anything related, you were tagged as a COVID patient, and the rest is history.

A lack of exercise or physical activity: it is true that exercise and physical activities improve the body's immune function and can reduce stress and our susceptibility to diseases. Sadly, most of us were indoors, which weakened our immune systems. Neutrophilis are a type of immune cell and the body's first line of defense against external microbes. They are like the police, patrolling our system and monitoring for invaders. When and if they detect a problem, they undergo chemotaxis, which involves engulfing or destroying the pathogen. Age lowers the efficacy of these immune fighters, but exercise or physical activities boost the T-cells and give you a fighting chance during an infection. This was clearly absent during the pandemic, and many seniors died because the simple stuff that helped them remain healthy was missing.

GOVERNMENT OVERSIGHT OR INTENTIONALITY?

Keeping the sun away from us was another controversy surrounding the lockdown. While the average American was asked to remain indoors, many elites were on a boat cruise, lounging in the sun and getting the best life at their expense. The sun helps coordinate our circadian rhythm, which enables you to sleep well, and without exposure to sunlight, the cells cannot function effectively or relate the information that the body needs. Additionally, being away from the sun meant spending more time behind the computer, absorbing the blue light that makes sleep difficult because the brain cells are active. The pandemic impacted our immune system and our psychology. It installed a fear of socializing and distrust among people, and how we responded to others increased our feelings of loneliness and state of wellness.

Moving on, contact tracing also meant that our personal space was invaded as the mobile smartphones of many people were tracked as we journeyed in our home environments or traveled abroad. In fact, some countries used malware to track contracts and for a variety of other purposes. Two or three years down the line, the lockdown and mandatory isolation regulations that restricted our mobility and deprived us of happiness and freedom did not really achieve their aim. Government officials and even Dr. Fauci have all admitted that we should learn to live with the virus and continue with our lives. Several studies across the world showed that the decision was terrible and did not reduce the mortality rate.

In extreme lockdown cases, the citizens' quality of life and happiness has changed. It does not really matter what you think; it is time we opened our eyes to see that our policymakers knew so little about the decisions they took to curb the virus' spread, including the lockdown.

THE PSYCHOLOGICAL COST OF CONTROVERSIAL LOCKDOWN AND QUARANTINE

Around one-third of the world's population, or around 2.6 billion people, are currently subject to some form of quarantine or lockdown. One may argue that this is the largest study of its kind ever done in the field of psychology.

We know what it will accomplish, and it won't be good. A analysis of 24 papers proving the psychological impact of quarantine (the "restricted of mobility of people who have potentially been exposed to a contagious disease") was published in The Lancet in late February 2020, just before European governments imposed various forms of lockdowns. These results provide a window into the daily lives of hundreds of millions of people all around the world.

In conclusion, and probably not unexpectedly, those who are quarantined are at a high risk of developing a wide range of symptoms of psychological stress and disorder, including poor mood, insomnia, stress, anxiety, rage, irritability, emotional weariness, melancholy, and post-traumatic stress symptoms. Particularly prevalent were low mood and irritation, the study found.

The first academic studies to examine the shutdown in China have already noted the anticipated mental health repercussions.

Isolating parents alongside their children also took a mental health toll. A minimum of 28% of quarantined parents met the criteria for a diagnosis of "trauma-related mental health problem" in one research.

Close to 10% of hospital employees who were sequestered experienced "strong depressed symptoms" up to three years after the end of their isolation. Long-term risks for alcohol misuse, self-medication, and long-lasting "avoidance" behavior were reported in another investigation evaluating the consequences of SARS quarantine on healthcare professionals. This means that even after being confined for a long period of time, some hospital staff members may still choose to avoid direct patient contact by not showing up to work.

There are several things that could cause stress during a lockdown, including the potential for infection, worries about getting sick or losing loved ones, and the possibility of financial difficulties. This current epidemic includes all of them and many more.

The second pandemic, and the erection of the virtual second tent

In countries that have gone into lockdown, we may already observe a dramatic rise in absenteeism. The fear of contracting COVID-19 on the factory floor has caused many people to stay home from work. In another three to six months, we'll see another swell of this. At a time when the economy needs as many hands as possible to fix it, we should expect a dramatic increase in absenteeism and burnout.

We know this from several real-world examples, such as the high rate of absenteeism among military units returning from deployment in high-risk locations, the businesses located near Ground Zero after 9/11, and the medical professionals who work in areas with Ebola, SARS, and MERS outbreaks.

These workers are likely to experience prolonged absences from the workplace as a result of health problems or exhaustion. Eurofound shows that even if these employees do remain on the job, their output drops by 35%.

Those working at the front lines of healthcare, people under the age of 30, children, the elderly, and those in vulnerable circumstances due to, among other things, mental illness, disability, or poverty are all known to be at increased risk for developing mental health problems over the long term.

All of this shouldn't come as a huge shock, given the science of trauma psychology has known for decades that tragedies have lasting effects.

However, the scope of these closures is unprecedented, even if the insights are not. A third of the world's population is struggling with these extreme stressors, so this time around ground zero is not a confined hamlet, town, or region. We must take immediate action to lessen the damage caused by this lockdown.

WHAT SCIENTISTS HAVE LEARNT FROM COVID CONTROVERSIAL LOCKDOWNS

It had been one year since the first wave of the COVID-19 pandemic prompted governments to implement the extreme measures commonly referred to as lockdowns. These included the cancellation of sporting and cultural events, the closure of stores, restaurants, schools, and universities, and the issuance of mandatory stay-at-home orders. There was a global outbreak of the coronavirus SARS-CoV-2 at the time, with different countries increasing or decreasing their lockdown policies in response.

Lockdown procedures were effective. Several studies showed that COVID-19 outbreaks might be reduced when people's social contacts were severely limited.

However, obstetrician and gynecologist Dr. Savaris from Porto Alegre's Federal University of Rio Grande do Sul and his colleagues conducted a new analysis (who worked in statistics, computer science and informatics). They used Google's anonymized mobile data to examine 87 areas around the world head-to-head to see if there was a correlation between a lower rate of COVID-19 mortality and more time spent at home. According to the findings of their study published in the journal Scientific Reports, it usually didn't.

Prominent shutdown skeptics and certain news outlets have brought attention to a number of academic publications, which have since become widely read. The results "were fairly astonishing, on the face of it," says Gideon Meyerowitz-Katz, an epidemiologist at Australia's University of Wollongong. He and others would prove that the paper's choice of statistical methods led to erroneous findings.

The journal Scientific Reports added a "editor's note" to the article within a week, informing readers of the criticisms. Two letters2,3 were published in the journal nine months later, detailing the paper's flaws. A week later, the paper was retracted, despite the fact that neither Savaris nor his co-authors agreed with the decision. (Springer Nature is the publisher of Scientific Reports, although the publication does not exert editorial control on Nature's reporting.)

Other studies have found that lockdowns did not prevent any deaths, therefore the retracted paper is not alone in its conclusion. However, these studies' analyses disagree with the vast bulk of research. Researchers agree that lockdowns reduced the number of individuals killed by COVID-19, and that governments were forced to limit social interactions in early 2020 to stop the spread of SARS-CoV-2 and prevent the collapse of healthcare systems. "We needed to give ourselves some time," UT Austin biological data scientist Lauren Meyers explains.

However, it is also obvious that lockdowns have substantial costs, and the value of any further lockout measures is open to question. There was disruption to education due to schools and universities being closed. Financial and social difficulties, as well as mental illness and economic downturns, were exacerbated as firms closed. Costs and advantages exist, argues public health statistician Samir Bhatt of Imperial College London and the University of Copenhagen.

Researchers have been analyzing the outcomes of lockdowns during the epidemic to better prepare for future emergencies. They have come to a few findings, such as the fact that nations who implemented tough policies first fared the best in terms of saving lives and maintaining economic growth. However, challenges have also been experienced by researchers. When weighing the costs and advantages of a situation, it's not always possible to use cold, hard math; instead, value assessments, including who should bear the brunt of the costs if some groups of people pay more than others, are often required. This makes lockdowns challenging to research and often fuels heated debate.

CRITICAL ASSESSMENT OF THE CONTROVERSIAL LOCKDOWN SITUATION

The analysis of the consequences of the COVID-19 lockdowns is complicated by the fact that it is difficult to know what would have happened if the lockdowns had not been implemented.

Shutting down Wuhan, China, after the initial outbreak of SARS-CoV-2 proved that lockdowns do limit viral transmission. Countries that didn't go as far as China and shut down their borders, tell their residents to remain home, and isolate those with COVID in central facilities nonetheless saw a reduction in disease transmission thanks to lockdown measures. For example, in May of 2020, Bhatt and coworkers analyzed lockdowns in 11 European countries, and based on the reduction in viral transmission, they concluded that the actions had saved more than 3 million lives.

The methods used in that section have also been called into doubt. One potential flaw is that the advantage may have been exaggerated due to the underlying assumption that people wouldn't have restricted their social contacts in the absence of lockdown mandates. Actually, people's actions would have been altered if death rates had been steadily climbing.

This implies that the US states' shelter-in-place orders had no effect on further reducing COVID-19 cases and deaths, not because social distancing doesn't work, but because people were already avoiding contact prior to the imposing of the orders.

Instead, some studies have tried to determine if countries with stronger lockdown rules fared better than those with more lenient ones on indicators like illness transmission rates and mortality rates. As if that weren't complicated enough, cultural context, population density, social contact, and virus prevalence all played a role in varying degrees of enforcement, amounts of government help, and conformity with official policies across regions.

Consider Sweden, which in early 2020 enacted comparatively mild limitations, allowing schools to remain open for all save the oldest kids. In 2020, its excess death rate was lower than that of many other western European countries. Because of its high levels of trust in government and the fact that many Swedes live alone (the country has the smallest average household size in the EU), the country has a lower rate of social contact and lower rates of disease transmission than other countries in the region. Instead of going about their typical activities, Swedes were less mobile than usual, as seen by their cell phone records. However, its Nordic neighbors that also instituted lockdowns fared better that year: data for Denmark, Finland, and Norway shows that their age-standardized mortality rates were lower than average in 2020, while those for Sweden show a modest increase over the previous year. (Like other countries, Sweden was unable to stop COVID-19 deaths among its most defenseless citizens, such as those in nursing homes for the elderly.)

3

FINDING A BALANCE – RESTRICTING THE PEOPLE'S LIBERTIES

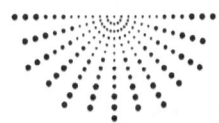

*T*he provision of public goods and the defense of civil freedoms are two of the state's primary functions. The state is committed to protecting civil liberties, including the right to due process, freedom of expression, and privacy, to the fullest extent practicable. According to political theorists, the major reason why people join a state and give up some independence is so that their remaining freedoms and rights can be better protected. Public goods, including safe air and effective law enforcement, are beneficial to society as a whole yet would be under-provided in a free market.

It's possible for the government's two primary responsibilities—protecting citizens' rights and providing essential services—to clash. For instance, in the name of ensuring national security, it's likely that people's private rights will be violated. Governments frequently have the challenging task of balancing competing demands and making difficult trade-offs.

These trade-offs become especially glaring at times of crisis, like as terrorist attacks and natural disasters, when protecting the public good may necessitate extreme measures that severely curtail human liberties.

One such example is the widespread spread of the COVID-19 virus. For the interest of public health, civil freedoms like freedom of movement and freedom of association, which had previously been virtually universally granted in democratic democracies, are being curtailed as part of the reaction to the pandemic.

Given the scope of the epidemic and the unprecedented steps taken by governments to contain it, the COVID-19 crisis presents a rare and terrible chance to learn how people feel about giving up their rights in exchange for better public health.

What will people give up in order to get through this catastrophe, and what will they stand by no matter what? How do the opinions of people in different countries and different subsets of a country's population differ from one another? How do these perceptions shift as the pandemic develops?

THERE ARE **at least three reasons why it's crucial that you answer the questions up top.**

IN A DEMOCRACY, first and foremost, the people's will should be reflected in the government's policies. Second, the level of public support for government responses to the pandemic will likely determine the extent to which those responses are followed. Third, the virus causes a wide range of symptoms, from no symptoms at all to life-threatening sickness and death; this diversity can increase polarization between those at risk and those who aren't, which can be harmful to the operation of democratic institutions.

Citizen perspectives from all over the globe

Our team conducted a large-scale representative survey among more than 400,000 people across 15 countries (Australia, Canada, China, France, Germany, India, Italy, Japan, the Netherlands, Singapore, Spain, South Korea, Sweden, the UK, and the US) to learn how people there feel about giving up some of their civil liberties in exchange for better public health during the COVID-19 pandemic. The study of the survey results led us to the following findings.

First, during the COVID-19 pandemic, many individuals all around the world said they were willing to give up some personal liberties in exchange for better public health. More than 80% of respondents reported being willing to compromise at least some of their own rights during a crisis like the current one, and this proportion rises to over 90% when we combine data from all the nations in our survey.

Core civil liberties were rated as important by respondents from all participating countries. People were not willing to give up things like privacy or democratically important activities in exchange for more personal constraints or financial losses.

There are significant disparities in opinion between nations; for example, people in Japan and the United States are among the least ready to give up personal freedoms in exchange for better public health. On the other hand, Chinese people appear to be among the most open. The average European Union resident probably isn't either extreme.

A Changing & Heterogeneous Willingness to Give Up Rights

The COVID-19 PANDEMIC HAS, in general, highlighted the tension between protecting individual liberty and protecting the public health. Our polling suggests that the vast majority of people everywhere would be ready to give up some privacy in exchange for better public health.

However, public support is likely to be diverse, depending on factors such as individuals' level of personal exposure to the health danger posed by COVID-19 and their concern about the potential infringement of their civil liberties. There are problems brought on by such divergent opinions since it becomes more difficult to reach compromise and consensus within individual nations.

Furthermore, as people's concerns about the health threats posed by COVID-19 lessened, so did their willingness to forgo their rights in reaction to the pandemic. It's possible that when health concerns decrease, public support and compliance with public health programs will also decline.

Concerns about civil liberties being eroded during the COVID-19 pandemic and a fluctuating willingness to give up rights over time emphasize that it is crucial to have robust safeguards that the regulations put in place during the pandemic would be turned back once the crisis is ended, and yet it is.

4

THE IMPACT OF THE CONTROVERSIAL LOCKDOWN ON COVID-19 SPREAD

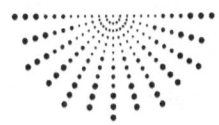

*T*he impact of the lockdown is still been felt across the world; the trauma and after-effect of the pain and inconsistency will forever remain a scar in families and history.

The COVID-19 lockdown debate is still ongoing as to whether the restrictive government measure was successful. A lockdown is a stay-at-home order to enable the government to track, trace, and curb an infection in the population. The claim is that the negative impact might outweigh the benefits because the economy, social life, education, and mental health of the citizen will be strongly affected. The controversy surrounding this claim is that the cure (the vaccine) was worse than the virus.

On January 23, 2020, China imposed the most drastic lockdown, shutting off over 11 million Wuhan residents from the outside world. The problem was a virus that would be listed among the deadliest pandemics of all time. Many called the COVID-19 lockdown the largest quarantine ever and this restricted human movement was to curb the spread and understand how the virus worked.

But did it work?

As human population grows, infection and infectious diseases are bound to happen with interactions across borders. Some left us marveling at their power to destroy, while others never knew when they happened. Either way, it was a learning experience, but the 2020 COVID-19 pandemic is not the first outbreak that demanded a lockdown (or, as in the days of old, a separation).

Lockdowns of the past

Human beings have suffered various plagues since the beginning of time. Whether by man-made mistake, nature, or some scientific mishap, these infections continue to garner strength and break human resolve every time they circle in. As diseases evolved with time, their impact was deadlier than the last. Additionally, human interaction with the unknown and animals in weird environments has left nothing to the imagination. Furthermore, the spread of diseases was also possible because more people clustered in city centers and had larger social circles.

So why is the pandemic so different, and why has it sparked so many controversies?

Some controversies relating to COVID-19 and the lockdown

When the population got wind of the outbreak late in 2020 and in the subsequent year, Wuhan was already on lockdown. This action would ultimately be the strategy to curb or subject people to a new normal on every continent. While the lockdown phenomenon is not new, as we have seen above, the COVID-19 strain of the virus left many, including scientists, in the dark. With no answer and mandatory policies, speculation filled the air, and many believed it.

The wearing of face masks

Facemasks were a mandatory action by the government to stop the spread of the virus, and while it was a cautionary measure until the workings of the virus were known, it sparked a wide controversy for many reasons. According to scientists, the virus was transmitted via droplets from speaking, coughing, and sneezing, and the facemask was mandatory to halt this. However, many questioned the effectiveness of the facemask in mitigating the spread. Some declared that this was only effective if physical distancing was in place. A clinical study revealed that while the mask prevented the spread of the virus, a face mask will not stop the wearer from inhaling small airborne particles, including the coronavirus.

If the facemask prevented the virus from getting into the mouth or nose, it did not stop it from getting into the eyes, triggering an itching sensation and an infection. If your hands are contaminated, you will therefore infect yourself even while wearing the facemask.

Hence, this preventive measure was unproductive if users touched their eyes in public.

Secondly, infected people, such as children, are less likely to wear a facemask in their homes, yet many parents interact with them. Furthermore, wearing a facemask prevented seamless breathing, making us breathe more deeply and often. This potentially moves the virus deep into the lungs, putting more people at risk if they have the virus.

The lockdown and immunity

For babies, infants, teens, and adults, interacting with our immediate surroundings and engaging in physical exercises build a strong immune system. This means getting fresh air, running in the park, getting dirty, and playing with their friends to mitigate stress, infections, and other developmental issues. With the pandemic lockdown, people couldn't enjoy activities or nature to boost their immune systems.

Did that make you susceptible to the virus?

We cannot overlook the use of hand sanitizer during the pandemic. Did it help? Many say yes, but are we missing the point? The idea of creating a sterile environment is impossible. Sanitized hands are the perfect surfaces for microbes and pathogens to dwell on via dust, air, supposedly clean surfaces, pets, objects in our surroundings, and many others. The truth is that while we desired to be clean, we also opened ourselves up to infection as crucial microbes were eliminated.

Immunologists are yet to decipher what is immune to the coronavirus looks or feels like. Studies on neutralizing antibodies show a high level of antibodies remains for weeks after infection before declining.

Does this mean the infected person can transmit the virus during recovery? Does it foil the effectiveness of the lockdown, and what are our chances of a lasting solution?

It is not difficult to see why the COVID-19 lockdown was followed by so many controversies. Many were worried about the health implications of being in a lockdown for extended periods (speaking on the immune system and the mental and emotional health of the citizens). Others argued about the economic downturn and the irreplaceable damage resulting from it. These and many more reasons explain why the global population resisted the lockdown because the government could not answer critical questions.

Additionally, many felt their human rights were truncated and their freedom limited.

World Health Organization (WHO) and the COVID-19 Lockdown

The WHO insisted that physical distance and stay-at-home orders would reduce the spread and ultimately kill the effect of the pandemic. However, these set measures did not achieve their true aim, and communities, societies, and nations around the world suffered immensely from the lockdown. For example: in many regions, the lockdown implied that there was no work or means to cater to you or your loved ones. Many people fell below the poverty line even in developed nations like the United States.

The World Health Organization chose this strategy to buy time while it understood the effects of the virus and how to start a vaccine process that did not follow all the proper procedures. Many applauded the organization for stepping up, but many described it as hypocritical and trying to use the pandemic as a way of depopulating the earth.

Aside from claiming that the virus was from a lab in Wuhan, what else do we really know about the pandemic that killed millions?

The Governments and lockdown

Throughout the history of disease and infections, one thing has been consistent: using quarantine practices to curb the spread of contagious diseases and minimize the death rate. Healthcare experts understand the significance of mitigating the impact, and COVID-19 is no different.

Quarantine or lockdown to curb the impact of the pandemic did not start today. This practice began in the 1300s as many cities suffered from the effects of the plague. The word "quarantine" originated in Italy and meant being secluded from the population for 40 days.

In 1918, the first pandemic of the 20th century was recorded. The spread was severe because of the First World War, but even more, the disease circulated among soldiers and other people using public transport and interacting with people daily. One safety measure implemented to curb the spread was to avoid large gatherings, stay indoors, and stop the media from propagating false information about the origin or capability of the virus. Even though these measures were not publicly announced, they sound familiar.

A hundred years later, we still implement the same lockdown strategies, with nothing learned from the century before. However, the laws are stricter, as people are banned from all public spaces, and safety measures, including disinfectants, sprays, and face covers, became the order of the day. The government also advocated physical distance to stop the spread.

Government and public health specialists across the world employed these restrictions, including mass testing and separation, for various reasons. While the governments of nations reacted differently to the pandemic in their respective countries, it also exposed the limitations of our government and the poor structure in place to fight the problem effectively. Yes, there were challenges, but the significant goals were to prevent the massive loss of lives as those recorded during past pandemics.

Did we achieve that? Well, it all depends on the point of view. Some of the challenges that made the COVID-19 lockdown confusing to many were:

The government's inability to accurately tell how the disease spread while denying people their fundamental freedom of movement rights was a miss. During the pandemic, it was not unusual to see people refusing to wear face-covering or keep a 6-foot distance apart. These negative externalities truncated people's liberty and put many others at risk of getting the disease.

The lack of factual medical data about the disease or solutions to cure it is another controversy surrounding the lockdown. This created a market for virus research, but the information was restricted to only those who could pay for it. Until now, Anthony Fauci has never really told the American people the genesis of vaccines or why specific labs were the first to produce them. Do we need to add that while the vaccine saved many lives, many more died from serious health complications related to the COVID-19 vaccine?

The irony is how we have moved ahead and forgotten the past so soon.

Are we waiting for the next pandemic mistake to tackle the gaps and damage to human lives? Did the lockdown really have such a massive impact on the spread? Regardless of your opinion, the government cannot justify its failures during the pandemic or deny that the violation of human rights produced the expected results.

THE GOVERNMENT FAILED **in many areas, including:**

PANDEMIC PREPAREDNESS: many nations lost tens of thousands of lives because the government did not anticipate the gravity and impending danger of the pandemic on their citizens. Basically, they failed to learn from other previous pandemics and lacked the capacities and knowledge to handle such an emergency in the 21st century. Additionally, pandemic preparedness includes risk management protocols, testing, and mitigation programs, as well as defining a standard that all medical personnel must follow to improve the problem and its impact.

Improper response to crisis management was another area where they failed woefully. For many, the government used the stay-at-home law to mask their inability to effectively manage their weak response or coordinate the right actors at various levels. This led to miscommunication, a lack of transparency, and distrust among the major players.

Poor response and recovery policies led to preventable deaths and losses for many individuals and families. The lockdown, though a restrictive measure to curb the spread, ignored the economic and welfare needs of the household. This meant people had to work to feed and cater to their families, making them more susceptible to infection and spreading it more.

To many people, the lockdown helped them manage the spread, but the harmful effect of the lockdown cannot be overlooked. The mandatory stay-at-home policy brought the nation and the world to a standstill, leading to high unemployment rates, discord in families, social isolation, and a huge loss to the economy.

The health, economic, and social issues are the biggest global impacts of the COVID-19 lockdown. There is a strain left by the lockdown, as countless people died or lost their livelihoods and relationships. While many grapple with returning to normalcy, mounting bills and a lack of work caused more severe health issues than many anticipated.

FEAR and psychological distress

COVID-19 triggered or enhanced mental issues in a great number of people. Many suffered from depression, anxiety, and fear or exhibited worrying behaviors, especially among healthcare workers. Fear was evident during the pandemic. For many, showing signs and symptoms of the disease meant a high chance of deformity or death and being away from family, as many people witnessed during the pandemic.

Additionally, young people felt isolated, socially distant, and disconnected in an uncertain world without school, friends, or activities to engage them. The lockdown also made domestic abuse, harassment, and molestation much easier to access. Women were not left out, as many experienced all forms of violence and suffered mental breakdowns during the first year of the pandemic.

. . .

Short-term mortality

The pandemic and the excessive lives lost were a rude awakening to a population for which death was always close by. For many, the death of a neighbor, parent, friend, or child made the tragedy so horrific. As many Americans are confronted with daily death numbers, we reflect on our own deaths. Additionally, the fear of dying also triggered pandemic-like symptoms in many and led to their untimely deaths. However, we cannot ignore the rude fact that the lockdown brought many people to a place of no control; we were at the mercy of the pandemic and what the government, media, and public health experts said. In the US, the death toll was choking as numbers rose daily, but the lack of concrete information on the pandemic and a cure for the virus was even scarier.

This short-term mortality was a deep fear as many people were separated from loved ones diagnosed with the virus. While the caregivers provided enough compassion and love to the patients, it would never be the same with their families. And as health workers interacted with infectious patients, they also spread the virus despite having access to the vaccine and safety amenities.

LACK OF ACCESS to health services and practitioners

The pandemic brought untold hardship to human life, as many people with various health challenges could not access health services. While the economic and social restrictions cannot be overlooked, many were at risk of dying without their regular medication or hospital visits. Although there is no concrete evidence of the spread due to restricted health access, the fear of many people coming into close contact with the disease might have put many people off. So they would rather stay home than attend healthcare centers for their problems.

INCREASED suicide rate and mental instability

The pandemic has had a severe impact on the mental health of individuals across the globe. While many suffered mental degradation due to unemployment and the inability to care for sick or un-sick loved ones, the lockdown was a fundamental trigger to suicidal thoughts. Whether suicide, self-harm, or suicidal thoughts, these are classified under the umbrella of mental health, which waned during the lockdown.

Additionally, because most people were indoors, sleep patterns changed, and adequate sleep and quality were reduced. The evidence suggests a strong link between sleep quality and mental health during the lockdown.

WHY DOES the COVID-19 Lockdown controversy still persist?

Confining the population to their homes reduced the spread; the concerns were whether the lockdown was truly mandatory without the necessary investigation and mitigation procedures. I hope readers will understand that the underlying cause and processes regarding COVID-19 were clearly missed from the outset, which led to the controversy.

I do not intend to complicate or exaggerate these issues, but rather to demonstrate why they continue to exist after two years.

When these lockdowns were issued by the government, it was a strategic approach to mitigate the spread of the virus. It was a preventive measure when the number of infections and deaths was at its barest minimum.

Unlike many countries worldwide, the USA is one that thoroughly investigates an issue and its impact on its citizens before taking any action that will affect them. The pandemic was different. The government and policymakers stamped out mandates without thoroughly analyzing the implications for its citizens. For example, while states ensured isolation, social distancing, reduced business time, facemasks, and fewer social gatherings, they failed to calculate the day-to-day activities of living.

The result was financial hardship, unemployment, and domestic issues in many homes across the country. It also resulted in people working odd jobs (because people had to eat and cater to loved ones), which meant interacting with people and being susceptible to the virus.

On the flip side, the public perceived the lockdown as the only way the government could control an uncontrollable situation laced with uncertainties and misinformation from the media and the government.

AFTER 2 YEARS, what are the negatives that still persist?

While the lockdown lasted, we cannot deny the amazing benefits it had on human lives, relationships, the environment, and our atmosphere. However, lawmakers should think thoroughly about any future lockdowns in the event of an outbreak, as some disastrous effects still linger.

We are still in the dark about COVID-19 and never anticipated the catastrophic effect the lockdown would have on society and people.

MASSIVE SPIKES in behavioral and mental issues

Crammed in a space for too long can have an untold impact on your psychology, and many people suffered during the lockdown. They had their social life taken from them and were prevented from interacting with friends, and family, or partaking in activities that elevated their suffering.

Even though, there was no 200% suicide rate as many claimed, <u>Trust for America's Health</u> reported the highest ever deaths during the COVID-19 pandemic from suicide, drugs and alcohol.

Drug and substance abuse

The lockdown created an avenue for people to indulge in habits intended to take away the mental impact of the lockdown. While many got productively busy, some others could not adapt to the process and depended on drugs to kill time. In many communities, drug intake doubled, mental instability spiked, and overdose deaths were recorded.

The inability of families to cater

Many people lost their jobs; we cannot forget the exponential numbers of parents and caregivers who lost their jobs due to the lockdown. As the country gradually returns to normalcy, the COVID-19 crisis has rendered many unable to feed or cater to their families. According to a <u>re-</u>

port in Wall Street Journal, many Americans cannot afford food for themselves of their families. In some households, many go hungry for days without any proper food. Additionally, food banks are reporting an increasing surge in demand, with malnutrition and starvation recorded in many communities.

DOMESTIC VIOLENCE, abuse, and oppression

Domestic violence and tension within the home were common news during the pandemic. People felt claustrophobic and cramped, crossing the boundaries of their partners. The problem is not restricted to developing countries but is rampant in developed nations too. Divorce rates also increased in several countries worldwide; from voluntary splits to separation, the pandemic put even the strongest relationships to the test. It was imminent, as sharing common spaces with the pressures of the lockdown was too much for some relationships to handle.

DID the government get it wrong?

Every country struggled during the pandemic and made disastrous mistakes that killed millions. China failed the world by not announcing the disease and silencing doctors, but it allowed a deadly virus to travel the world. Countries in Europe were, for the most part, lackadaisical. They ignored warning signs until it was too late, and the death toll was too high to count. The US also failed in many ways.

Many countries that looked to the US were disappointed as the pandemic became a political toy for the elite. Regardless of what happened, the pandemic clearly showed that no one country can solve the problem of an outbreak alone.

WHERE DID the US miss it?

WHITEWASHING the dangers of the virus

This was a significant reason the virus spread like wildfire—the government's attempt to sideline experts and make it a laughable stock. Then President Trump waved the virus off as no worse than the flu. Additionally, his administration's limited information and health data stopped the

CDC from appropriately doing its job and had the backing of the media on the charade that it would be over by Easter; apparently, it did not happen, and millions lost their lives.

Flaws and Inconsistent Testing Approach

The facts are undeniable: The CDC could not produce the massive testing kits needed to conduct the swift testing necessary to combat the spread of the coronavirus. Additionally, their supposedly reliable test was flawed, producing inaccurate results, yet permission for efficient companies dragged on, causing preventable deaths. For the most part, testing was unevenly distributed, and the virus and infected individuals were rampant, thwarting the efficacy of the lockdown.

Slow tracing, isolating, and quarantining method

Pandemics of the past showed that efficient and swift tracing, isolation, and quarantine were the most effective measures to combat a spread, especially since little was known about COVID-19.

Although the World Health Organization reiterated the significance of this process, many countries were in over their heads and lost track of the virus's movement.

Finally, the battle for proper COVID-19 guidance and the delivery of information was slow and irregular for the most part.

WHERE ARE WE TODAY?

We live amid a pandemic with so many strains that we have almost lost count. We are just waiting for the health experts to announce the latest mutations or variants. However, we must also not forget that despite the variants, people are going about their business and not keeping with the COVID-19 rules. Many people have forgotten about facemasks or being six feet apart.

Hopefully, the world gets to herd immunity and the virus disappears like past pandemics, but caution is the watchword for safety. Today, the vaccine is still undergoing testing, and better options to curb the disease are available to anyone.

The future is bright, even though scientists think it will never leave and the human body will develop immunity over time. COVID-19 remains a mystery, and someday, just maybe, we will read about the real truth in the pages of a science journal.

FINAL THOUGHT

The lockdown will remain controversial, as the government or public health experts could not answer the many questions its citizens asked during the pandemic. Additionally, the secrecy and flood of misinformation left little to be desired about the scenario. Several times, stories from across the world told about how patients without COVID-19 symptoms were treated as having the disease, even before proper testing. Furthermore, with information about doctors being paid to inject patients or count non-COVID deaths as COVID deaths, we could only imagine. Even if our healthcare system failed due to unpreparedness, the WHO did not deliver on its mandate to protect and provide adequate care. Some say it is politics; others say the global elites have their hands in it to reduce the world population.

After reading through countless COVID stories and studies on the topic, it is not unsound to accept the controversies that surround the lockdown or its effectiveness in curbing the spread. There were people that never wore the facemask and had an active social life, refused the vaccines and never got infected. Yet, many followed the order, got the virus, got the vaccine and died.

Whether you believe the government was right or not, the pandemic was a social experiment for a probable health event in the future. To all those who believe what the government and public health experts said,

I have a question for you. Why haven't the government answered questions on the whys, hows, when, what and where?

Why are we still in the dark until today? The world should know these data so that they can work together and take the necessary steps to prevent the spread of another deadly virus that might annihilate the human race.

What can we say? If nobody was booked for the virus that killed millions around the globe, then there is a story that is being protected from the world.

Did the lockdown combat the spread of the coronavirus? Many people think it helped but it also caused many other problems that could be preventable.

That in itself is a controversy that needs answers.

5

LIMITED TRUST - VACCINES BIG PHARMA COOPERATION

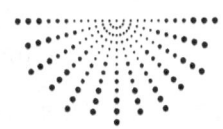

*O*ver the decades leading up to the Covid-19 epidemic, Big Pharma had been gradually withdrawing from the vaccination market. In 2019, only a small number of conglomerates including Merck, Sanofi, Pfizer, and Johnson & Johnson remained as significant suppliers of vaccines to the United States. Vaccines are not lucrative because they are only used once or twice, unlike regular medications. Due to their widespread implementation, vaccination programs can easily become the target of class action lawsuits.

The Obama administration required a massive sum of money to convince pharmaceutical firms to invest in research and testing, and then to create hundreds of millions of doses. Ten billion dollars was first requested, and it was promptly appropriated by Congress. U.S. government's Covid-19 alleviation scheme, "Operation Warp Speed" (OWS), will ultimately give $22 billion to Big Pharma.

The quantities of money involved were enormous for a public health endeavor, with Moderna receiving $2.5 billion, AstraZeneca $1.2 billion, Johnson & Johnson receiving $500 million, and a little business called Novavax receiving $1.6 billion. Pfizer was the lone company that first declined to contribute to the trough because it was unwilling to spend time and money working in tandem with the United States government.

One hundred million doses of Pfizer's two-shot vaccine were sold to the United States for $1.95 billion in July, enough to protect fifty million individuals. It would arrive at American weapons first. A double dose costs about as much as a single dose of the flu vaccine. Due in part to the United States' nearly a billion dollar investment in Moderna research, the government had ordered three hundred million doses from the company by February, with the first shipment of one hundred million costing thirty dollars per double-shot dose, cheaper than Pfizer. The CEO of Moderna has stated that once government contracts are no longer in place, the retail price per dose will increase.

The project's success makes it unlikely that its finances will be scrutinized.

Pharmaceutical business executives and their political allies staffed OWS at all levels. Thanks to a specific exemption, they may keep their investments if they so desired. Since they were hired as "contractors," federal conflict-of-interest regulations that apply to employees did not apply to them. OWS advisors with investments and ties were required to agree to assign a portion of their future profits from the Covid vaccine to the NIH, though this could occur only after their deaths.

Moderna and Pfizer executives made millions off the vaccine by selling stock just before news of positive clinical study results was made public.

Pharmaceutical business executives and their political allies populated OWS at every level. A specific exemption allowed them to keep their investments if they so chose. Since they were hired on as "contractors," they were exempt from federal conflict-of-interest restrictions that apply to regular workers. OWS advisors with investments and ties were required to agree to assign a portion of their future profits from the Covid vaccine to the NIH, though this could occur only after their deaths.

Moncef Slaoui, formerly of Big Pharma, served on the board of Moderna. According to Securities and Exchange Commission papers, originally examined by Kaiser Health News, Slaoui was granted options to purchase 18,270 shares in the company on March 13, just 13 days after the first big inflow of government money into its coffers, which prompted a rise in the stock price. These were in addition to the 137,168 choices he had already amassed as of 2018. When he left the board of Moderna, he walked away with an estimated $8 million.

William Erhardt and Rachel Harrigan, both Pfizer employees and OWS advisers, kept undisclosed financial stakes in the company that awarded them a nearly $2 billion deal for 100 million doses of their vaccine. Vaccine safety panel member and Gilead employee Richard Whitley is also involved with the company that makes the antiviral drug, Remdesivir, which is distributed by Covid. Carlo de Notaristefani, a Trump adviser, has ties to Teva, the manufacturer of hydroxychloroquine. Dr. Mark McClellan, a former FDA commissioner, and Dr. Scott Gottlieb, a former FDA commissioner, both serve on the boards of Covid vaccine makers and provide informal advice to the federal response.

Insiders who traded on the company's good news made even more money. Vaccine executives at Moderna and Pfizer sold stock in the company at the exact moment that news of positive clinical trial results was released to the public.

Stock transactions at such inopportune times are neither uncommon nor prohibited. Economist Joshua Mitts of Columbia Law School showed that executives in a wide variety of industries are up to three times more likely to sell o their company stock on days when their companies disclose great news than on days when negative, neutral, or no news is provided.

Pfizer CEO Albert Bourla sold 62% of his holdings on November 9 after the company claimed a vaccination efficacy of more than 90%. The stock market reacted favorably to the news, sending prices soaring by 15%. Equilar, a provider of executive remuneration and corporate governance statistics, informed the Los Angeles Times that Bourla was one of seven Pfizer executives who received a combined $14 million via stock transactions in 2020.

Moderna's top brass earned $287 million in 2020 from well-timed stock transactions and continued right on working. Moderna CEO Stéphane Bancel disposed out millions of dollars' worth of shares in a matter of days in late January and early February 2021.

One of the most ambitious attempts in the Trump administration's free market ideological playbook is the Covid solution, which involves throwing public money at private enterprise with essentially little oversight of the contracting system. The whole lineup of this pharmaceutical windfall club will probably never be published.

Governments may have exploited the pandemic crisis as an opportunity to restructure the 1980s-era shareholder model of for-profit medicine, which prioritized profits over public health. Instead, taxpayer dollars went to a select number of capitalists with virtually no oversight or accountability. Although Freedom of Information Act

(FOIA) requests have been filed, the contracts have been redacted.

A few of the researchers were sought out and lauded as heroes by the media as vaccinations were implemented in cities across the country at the end of 2020. And it is true that they are heroes. Most scientists, though, would pass up the opportunity to cash in. Barney Graham, whose research at the NIH on molecular protein manipulation was important in the development of the Moderna vaccine, is a government employee. Moderna executives will continue charge the United States for its vaccination while taking home nearly a billion dollars.

The University of Pennsylvania, not the Hungarian biochemist Katalin Karikó, owns the patent on her work that was instrumental in creating the BioNTech-Pfizer vaccine. However, Ugur Sahin and zlem Türeci, the company's cofounders, have made a lot of money. The married physicians pictured at the top are now billionaires and among the wealthiest people in Germany. In 2016, they made a $1.4 billion sale of their pharmaceuticals company, Ganymed.

The United States spent $18 billion on vaccine development, production, and distribution in 2020, and by year's end, two vaccines—those developed by Pfizer and Moderna on the mRNA platform—had been given the green light for usage. The eleven-month timeline from first idea to emergency approval was a first in the United States vaccine industry. There really was no competition.

In addition to the mRNA vaccines, the US government had invested heavily in Johnson & Johnson, Novavax, and the British pharmaceutical firm AstraZeneca. Using a virus engineered so that it can enter cells but cannot proliferate, pharmaceutical giants Johnson & Johnson and AstraZeneca were developing vector vaccines, a newer vaccination model than the attenuated viral model popular since the days of the cowpox. The vector vaccines inject disease-specific genetic information into cells using viruses already present in the body (often the common cold-causing adenovirus).

6

VACCINE LIBERTY—THE PEOPLE'S CHOICE

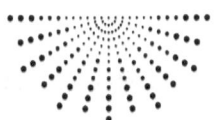

*Y*ou could have read interview pieces or heard from a friend or neighbor that you shouldn't receive the COVID-19 vaccine since it's "experimental."

It highlights the fact that even after more than 27 months of a pandemic, with 1 in 545 Americans dying from COVID-19, a sizable minority of the population continues to choose personal freedoms over the greater good.

At a pivotal time when partisan factionalism and social media are both accomplishing identical goals, this huge division — which has spread into businesses, schools, supermarkets, and voting booths — has separated the nation.

It's a phenomenon that leaves philosophers, scientists, lawyers, and experts in public health wondering:

When do private interests have to give way to the common good? Can we expect a shift in opinion if 1 out of every 100 people die from coronavirus? Or 1 in 10?

Millions of people in the United States today passionately oppose government regulations and refuse to get immunizations despite their demonstrated efficacy or wear protective masks.

Others want for stricter rules, saying people who don't take care are endangering the lives of everyone around them.

According to research from Johns Hopkins University, COVID-19 is now responsible for over 2,000 deaths each week in the United States, and the number of new infections has risen beyond 60,000 per day for the first time in over three months. In the words of the U.S. Centers for Disease Control and Prevention, nearly two-thirds of the nation's counties are struggling with substantial or high transmission rates.

This setting has given rise to an apparent contradiction: Today, over 99 percent of Americans who die from COVID-19 did not receive vaccinations. The unvaccinated, who are at a higher risk of contracting and spreading the disease, also tend to be the least likely to take precautions such as wearing a mask.

Despite the fact that scientific understanding is still developing and medical messaging has been muddied, the vaccination has proven to be highly effective.

So, vaccinations really do save lives.

And since vaccines have the potential to halt the spread of the virus, they might also speed up the recovery of the economy and social order. Why, therefore, do so many refuse vaccinations and refuse to use protective gear? Does this person have a social disorder where they prioritize their own needs over those of society as a whole? Can it be called a principled stance? Is there another explanation?

Although hiding one's identity by wearing a mask is simple, those who are against them are motivated by a different worry: they don't want the government telling them how to live their lives.

The opposition, however, is not motivated by concerns for public health; rather, "it's about politics."

The pandemic's emphasis on our interdependence is countered by the stunning lack of unity and shared sacrifice it has prompted. No one was ready for the epidemic, not just on a practical and medical level, but also on a moral one. It came at the worst possible time, when social relationships were already strained and the political climate was poisonous.

Not out of any sense of self-interest, but rather as a statement of moral outrage, they refuse to accept scientific evidence and defy authority. And that attitude is bolstered by the online community that serves as an echo chamber for the disenfranchised.

Unfortunately, COVID-19 lacks a political philosophy and an ethical compass. More than 4.2 million people have died around the world because the virus has spread so rapidly, especially among individuals who didn't obtain vaccinations.

In the UK, vaccines and other medical procedures typically require informed permission from the patient. This is not unique to the coronavirus vaccine.

Medical treatment can be administered against your will only in very specific circumstances, such as those outlined in the Mental Capacity Act 2005 (which governs the care and treatment of those who lack the mental capacity to make such decisions for themselves) and the Mental Health Act 1983 (which governs the treatment of those who are detained).

Except under these limited circumstances, it is a violation of your human rights and international medical treaty obligations to be coerced into receiving a vaccination. This means that you cannot be coerced into getting the vaccine unless you lack the mental capacity to give your informed permission.

7

COVID-19 POLITICS – WHO CALLED THE SHOTS?

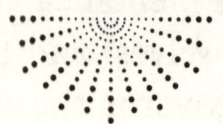

ost Americans lack the ability to independently investigate a topic. For the most part, people wouldn't understand what they read even if they performed their own investigation.

This meant they have to rely on others to do the legwork and draw any conclusions.

As a result, they are forced to rely on the decisions made by the government. Regrettably, government employees lack scientific training. They are both equally unable to understand academic journal articles. What good does it do to live in a country like the United States if the president picks someone obviously incapable of leading the country's efforts to improve its citizens' psychological and physiological well-being?

The government tries to persuade the public that the Covid vaccination is the best choice by excessively politicizing the issue. But the government is a monolith with no room for individual preferences. Any suggestions for change from citizens will be disregarded by the administration. All citizens will be pressured by the government to conform to that one option. Those who opt for different approaches must then consider political factors.

Two explanations can be offered for the politicization of Covid vaccinations. Here are the two main ones. On an episode of Neil deGrasse Tyson's StarTalk, a sociologist who analyzes historical responses to epidemics and plagues provided one possible explanation. It turns out that this is just how people are; when one group prepares to combat a perceived threat to public health, the more traditional group tends to act in a more tribal fashion. It's happened during every public health crisis we've had, and in other events like the fight to enforce seat belts and so on. If one group in society declares, "we want this because we want this," then another group will always find a way to resist.

The other, and more important, reason for the severity of this one, is that conservatives in our political system have learned that anger and hatred are more effective than other messages when appealing to their base. You may see this theme repeated in the conservative drive to rebuild the party after Nixon's departure brought party humiliation, as well as in the "Those Angry Days" buildup to WWII and the conservative buildup to the Civil War. If you recall, the drive for "save our babies" started shortly after that, leading to the first abortion center bombings and so on. The politicization of the reaction to the COVID outbreak is only the latest example of conservatives capitalizing on the fears and anger of their constituents.

It's not uncommon for scientific findings to be manipulated for broader political, economic, or cultural purposes. When people ignore good scientific advice because it's politically incorrect, the politicization of research dampens the potential benefits of scientific progress. There is little question that the politicization of this issue has influenced people's reluctance to use the COVID-

19 vaccine. In order to increase the use of life-saving vaccines, it is urgent for scientists and clinicians to better understand (1) the origins of politicization in regards to COVID-19 vaccines, (2) the factors that influence people's receptivity to scientific misinformation in politicized contexts, and (3) how to combat the politicization of science. Concerning the rise of vaccine-resistant COVID-19 in the USA, this chapter delves into these questions. Following a brief overview of vaccine research, we discuss how the disease was politicized in response to statements made by political leaders and reported in the media, particularly on social networking sites.

We then examine the politics of the vaccination on a global scale, the variation in public acceptability of the vaccines in the United States, and the response to the development of variations. Following this, we provide a synopsis of the social science literature on overcoming vaccine resistance, and last, we discuss the implications of the politicization of the disease and vaccination for medical professionals and biomedical researchers.

. . .

How Did the COVID-19 Virus Itself Become Politicized?

When political identities or cues become integrated into public discourse, this is called "politicizing" a health-related issue. One example is when the media highlights a political debate on a topic, leading some people to acquire biased opinions when presented with new scientific evidence. Partisan divides in public discourse about vaccination and media coverage about the biology of the virus all contributed to the politicization of COVID-19 vaccinations.

1. Prominent Politicians' Statements & The CDC's Use of Visual Cues

At first, President Trump minimized the seriousness of COVID-19 by comparing it to the flu. He also said that "the Democrats are politicizing the coronavirus—they're politicizing it," calling it a "new scam." The President has also advocated for the use of hydroxychloroquine as a treatment and has supported the idea that the virus can be neutralized by injecting or ingesting disinfectant or bleach. Similarly, he made public appearances without a mask while mocking his competitor for the presidency, Joe Biden, for wearing one: "Did you ever see a man that likes a mask as much as him?... To paraphrase a psychiatrist: "This guy has some serious problems."

To put it another way, partisanship was "built into the context of the emergent coronavirus... From the early warning, Republican lawmakers followed Trump's lead in publicly downplaying the threat, while Democrats responded with more concern, exhibiting different public signs." Furthermore, President Trump's tweets implying or that unproven remedies should be employed persuaded certain members of the American public to think so.

The Centers for Disease Control and Prevention (CDC) is the principal organization "known as the nation's top health promotion, prevention, and preparedness agency" in the United States. Since its inception in 1946, this agency's research on both communicable and non-communicable diseases has made important contributions to improving public health across the country. During the COVID-19 epidemic, the FDA sent conflicting messages to the public about the severity of the disease and how to avoid contracting it. That agency's "connection to disease control had shifted in ways that undercut its need for daring," as Michael Lewis put it. It was already falling. The house had swapped out the real flowers on the front porch for fake ones and thought no one would notice. "Unquestionable record was tainted by technical mistakes, lack of leadership, and inconsistent signals throughout the pandemic," as Guharoy and Krenzelok put it, "by the CDC." They point to things like the government's inability to supply a COVID-19 test kit at the start of the pandemic and the likelihood that it caved to pressure from the Trump administration "to encourage the use of invalidated treatments."

Representatives from both parties in the United States House of Representatives requested a report from the Select Subcommittee on the Coronavirus Crisis, and its staff found 47 instances of government interference, including "repeatedly overruling and sidelining top scientists and undermining Americans' health to advance the President's partisan agenda." The CDC travel notice was delayed, plans to distribute reusable masks to every household in the United States in April 2020 were halted, shutdown orders were lifted, and scientific reports on the nature of the virus were delayed or censored due to political influence.

2. Reports in the Media

Since the pandemic began, multiple news outlets have spread conflicting party rhetoric. For instance, a number of mainstream conservative media outlets have argued that the virus poses less of a concern to public health than has been made out. Instead, some argued that the media's emphasis on the severity of the virus was exaggerated, that the Chinese government was behind the attempt to undermine the US economy, or that the "deep state" was behind the effort to sow fear and damage Trump's re-election prospects. Fox News was much more likely than CNN or MSNBC to use words raising suspicion about the implications of the COVID-19 outbreak, such as "regular flu," "political weapon," and "flu hysteria," during the outbreak's whole (February 1, 2020 - April 30, 2020).

The politicization of the virus was exacerbated by posts on social media. False claims (such that coronavirus is transferred through mosquito bites) and conspiracy theories (5G towers are spreading the virus) together with pseudoscientific health cures gained widespread attention on social media (eating garlic or drinking bleach can cure the disease). This epidemic of misinformation on social media has been called a "misinfodemic" because of how quickly and widely it has spread.

3. Partisan Disparities in Response

Without a vaccine, governments tried other measures to reduce the spread of the illness, including "social distancing," the closure of schools and other public facilities, remote work, limits on public gatherings, quarantines, hand washing, and the use of masks. The success of these NPIs, like that of immunizations, was impacted by party differences in the perceived gravity of the illness and desire to comply with NPIs as a result of politicization in media coverage and communication via social media.

POLITICIZATION of the COVID-19 Vaccine

Some members of the public may be more receptive to false information about COVID-19 vaccines due to the debate in the political sphere and media coverage of the virus's existence and potential dangers. It has been suggested that people's feelings about becoming vaccinated can be "conceived as a continuum ranging from outright refusal to active demand for immediate uptake."

Since the initial phases of testing for COVID-19 vaccines, polls suggested that a large percentage of people in the United States were vaccine resistant, characterized as refusing to become vaccinated once one became available. Vaccine hesitancy can be characterized as the desire to wait until others have made the decision for you before making your own. Vaccine resistance or reluctance has varied throughout time and has been affected by factors such as knowledge, the state of the epidemic, and personal traits.

• DISCUSSION of the processes involved in creating and approving vaccines

. . .

ON MAY 15, 2020, President Trump announced Operation Warp Speed, a public-private partnership with $10 billion in financing from Congress to facilitate faster development and approval of a vaccine for COVID-19. This, Trump said, would be "a gigantic scientific, industrial, and logistical operation unlike anything our country has seen since the Manhattan Project," and it would have to be accomplished "large and it would have to be accomplished fast." The major objective was to "develop and deliver 300 million doses of safe and effective vaccinations, with the initial doses available by January 2021," as stated by the Department of Health and Human Services. By doing so, the government helped pharmaceutical firms manufacture and store approved vaccines, coordinated with other federal agencies, and sped up the process of developing new vaccines. However, there was already a lot of misunderstanding about COVID-19 vaccinations, and "a more hazardous environment for science communication is hard to imagine: a novel vaccine, possibly fast-tracked, in the middle of a highly political and badly mishandled epidemic." The anti-vaccine movement was undoubtedly helped by the Trump administration's choice of term for this project, which made it easy to portray COVID-19 vaccine studies as putting speed ahead of safety. "I'm a little troubled by that name because it can imply... that you're running so fast that you're skipping over crucial processes and not paying enough attention to safety," said National Institute of Allergy and Infectious Diseases Director Anthony Fauci.

Media coverage of the safety and effectiveness of any emergency-authorized COVID-19 vaccines was heavily influenced by the conflict and the partisan implications of immunizations, as Operation Warp Speed occurred during the US presidential campaign and election. Concern that "political forces" like the U.S. presidential election on November 3, nationalistic pride to "win" a race, and the need to "resuscitate economies" could lead to "premature and dangerous approvals...by the U.S. Food and Drug Administration" stemmed from the fact that China and Russia had been heavily criticized for authorizing emergency use of COVID-19 vaccines outside of clinical trials.

President Trump also said that getting emergency approval for a COVID-19 vaccination before Election Day would enhance his prospects of re-election. An story in The New York Times expressed fear that the FDA would speed through the approval of a vaccination in order to appease the President. Moreover, the vaccine sparked political disputes over the merits of mandatory vaccinations, fears of "immunization cards" that people would be obliged to carry, and a loss of individual rights by allowing government to regulate personal health decisions. The public's faith in the vaccine's safety and their intents to get vaccinated were dampened by the politics of the approval process and the possibility that the vaccine would be released before the election.

China, Russia, and the United States all competed to be the first to market a successful vaccine, which stoked national-level politics surrounding vaccine development. This was blamed on "vaccine nationalism" by official bodies and major media outlets. Examining the Global Times (China) and the New York Times (USA) for their respective coverage of vaccine development, Abbas discovered that the former launched "a misinformation campaign against American vaccines," while the latter cast doubt on the reliability and efficacy of the Chinese Sinovac vaccine.

· · ·

• Immune Response Variability

Concern, opposition, and sharply divided opinions all stem from the politicization of COVID-19 vaccinations. In June of 2020, surveys indicated that only 34% of Americans would be willing to get vaccinated against COVID-19, with strong partisan differences. Voters who supported Trump in the election were 35% less likely to report getting the COVID-19 vaccine. The percentage of Americans planning to get vaccinated increased as vaccine availability grew in the spring of 2021, yet it remained lowest among Republicans. Partisanship is a significant influence of sentiments regarding the pandemic and self-reported behaviors, as stated by Allcott et al.

A higher percentage of Republicans, compared to Democrats, believed false information about the dangers of vaccines. The growth of right-wing populist themes that pit "ordinary people" against "corrupt elites" may have contributed to this increased distrust of the scientific community among conservatives. The rejection of scientific statements about vaccines has been linked to a general distrust of specialists. 58 Conservatives may have been less receptive to public health messages because populist rhetoric conditioned them to value emotion over reason.

High levels of polarization can be traced back to people's reliance on the opinions and recommendations of influential elites. In late March 2021, for instance, researchers compared the impact of showing people either President Joe Biden's or Former President Donald Trump's short videos and statements advocating COVID-19 vaccines.

In a test with a control group, Republicans who heard a vaccine message from Trump were more inclined to say they would be vaccinated than those who heard the same message from President Biden, the out-party leader.

The observed belief polarization after exposure to identical signals from opposing ideological elites may have been driven by disparities in the perceived reliability of partisan sources, even among individuals seeking factual information. One important takeaway is that unvaccinated Republicans are more likely to accept a COVID-19 vaccine after being exposed to a pro-vaccination message endorsed by a Republican leader, and that people's underlying goals or motives shift between situations.

A study found that people in locations with higher degrees of polarization were more inclined to conform with others of their in-group regarding health-behavior responses to the COVID-19 issue, indicating that people tend to share the views of their neighbors.

Individuals' biases in evaluating scientific arguments, evidence, and political information shape their decision-making and information processing. COVID-19 was "a illness that quickly got politicized in the United States," and people in these situations are especially susceptible to vaccine disinformation because they are more likely to rely on identity affirmation than on a rigorous review of data. People are often motivated to evaluate new information in a way that protects their prior beliefs, worldviews, and social identities due to the importance of "identity affirmation" in the processing of scientific information; for example, they may seek out information that supports their existing views when forming beliefs and making decisions (confirmation bias), or they may avoid or argue against information that challenges an existing belief or identity (prior attitude effect).

Furthermore, the politicization of the vaccine intertwined with the proliferation of vaccine conspiracy theories. Conspiracy theories are unproven explanations for events in which an individual or group of individuals engage in deception that is damaging to others for their own gain. Conspiracy theories about COVID-19 have blamed many parties, including "China, Russia, Bill Gates, Democrats, the 'deep state,' and the pharmaceutical business, to mention a few." Conspiracy theories backed by partisan figures had a greater impact on audiences' levels of misunderstanding about COVID-19 than medical disinformation concerning the virus's transmissibility, according to a national study of US adults conducted in June 2020. Conspiracy theorists tend to be less open to scientific information, more receptive to the politicization of science, and less likely to engage in prosocial health practices, especially on matters where there is politicization and party polarization.

8

PURSUING A NATURAL SOLUTION

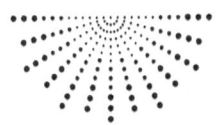

*N*atural remedies for COVID-19 have been proven effective in clinical trials.

They discovered that the natural compounds in green tea, olive oil, and red wine can block a major coronavirus enzyme; that moderate exercise for just 150 minutes per week can reduce the risk of contracting coronavirus; that eating ultra-processed foods is linked to severe viral infection; that nicotine has been shown to have cytoprotective activity against a pandemic; and that making out can improve cardiovascular health, alleviate sinus congestion, and ward off COVID-19.

Chemical substances can shield cells from damage through a mechanism called cytoprotection.

Actually, green tea, olive oil, and red wine have three natural chemicals that show promise as potential therapeutic ingredients against the coronavirus.

The compounds were identified by a systematic screening of a huge library of natural chemicals using DESY's X-ray source PETRA III, where the compounds were found attached to a key enzyme essential for the replication of the coronavirus.

Hamburg, Germany is home to the Deutsches Elektronen-Synchrotron (DESY), a Helmholtz Association Research Center. After being put into service in 2009, PETRA III quickly became the most powerful X-ray radiation source in the world based on the use of storage rings.

The highest intensity X-ray source, it provides researchers with unprecedented access to cutting-edge experimental possibilities. Small-sample researchers and those needing highly collimated, short-wavelength X-rays will benefit the most from this.

The group led by Christian Betzel from the University of Hamburg and Alke Meents from DESY writes in the journal Communications Biology that all three compounds are already utilized as active ingredients in existing medications. However, it is yet to be determined whether or whether these chemicals can form the basis of a medication against coronaviruses.

According to the study's lead author, University of Hamburg researcher Vasundara Srinivasan: "We evaluated 500 compounds from the Karachi Library of Natural Compounds if they bind to the papain-like protease of the novel coronavirus, which is one of the key targets for an antiviral medication. Inhibition of an enzyme's activity can be achieved by binding a specific chemical to it.

Virus replication requires the papain-like protease (PLpro): Coronaviruses are notorious for their ability to take over host cells and push them to make replica copies of the virus. Proteins are typically produced in the form of a lengthy strand in the lab. Following this, PLpro operates like a molecular pair of scissors to separate the proteins from the thread. If the proteins are prevented from completing this step, they will be unable to form new virus particles.

As Srinivasan pointed out, "However, PLpro has another crucial function for the virus. It inhibits an immune system protein known as ISG15, which significantly reduces the cell's ability to defend itself. By blocking PLpro, we can boost the immunological response of the cell.

Each of the five hundred natural compounds was dissolved alongside PLpro in a solution and tested for its ability to bind to the enzyme. Using a regular light microscope, you can't tell if something binds to the enzyme or not. Instead, the combinations were used to cultivate microscopic crystals. Crystals were exposed to intense X-rays from PETRA III at the P11 experimental station, resulting in a distinctive diffraction pattern that allowed the enzyme's atomic structure to be reconstructed.

To combat the ongoing epidemic, researchers have developed a number of vaccinations, treatments, and non-pharmaceutical measures to counteract COVID-19. However, people would be better able to prevent future SARS-CoV-2 infections if they knew more about the risk factors linked with infection.

The quality of one's diet is widely acknowledged as a crucial factor in maintaining good health. An key element in immunological regulation, a healthy gut microbiota is linked to eating a balanced diet.

A decreased risk of contracting COVID-19 was seen in people who ate more fruits and vegetables and otherwise followed a healthy plant-based diet. This finding may suggest that COVID-19 and diet are connected.

The NOVA classification system divides products with food as their base into four distinct categories, each of which is defined by the level and goal of industrial processing. Ultra-processed foods (UPFs) are the most processed of the four categories, consisting of industrial formulations of refined food ingredients such fats, oils, starches, sugars, and protein isolates. These foods go through chemical processes such as hydrogenation, hydrolysis, or the addition of dyes, flavors, and emulsifiers.

Extremely processed foods (UPFs) are notorious for their obscene amounts of unhealthy fats, sugars, trans fats, and salt. They also have a negligible amount of protein, fiber, vitamins, and minerals.

The composition of the gut microbiota and the risk of inflammation may be affected by UPFs, which have been shown in multiple studies to be a major dietary source of food adulterants and neo-formed chemicals.

Those who rely excessively on UPF-rich diets may be at risk for mineral and vitamin deficiencies, immune system damage, and illness. Inflammatory bowel illness, cardiovascular disease, and cancer are all more likely to occur in people with UPFs.

Insufficient data exist to draw conclusions on whether or whether consuming UPF raises the chance of contracting COVID-19, according to scientists. In light of this knowledge vacuum, researchers in a study published in the European Journal of Nutrition looked into possible links between UPF intake and the spread of SARS-CoV-2.

9

REFLECTING ON THE PANDEMIC

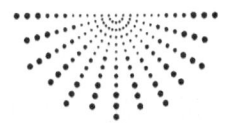

The coronavirus has drastically altered human society. Our lives were turned upside down as the 21-day lockdown lasted for months, then a year, and finally beyond what anyone could have predicted. We experienced historic shifts, such the elimination of the 10th boards, and began to enjoy the benefits of remote employment and online education.

While the terror of COVID-19 paralyzed us, it also provided a fresh perspective on the world. We've all gone through phases where we try to satisfy our hunger by cooking elaborate meals, like Dalgona coffee with banana bread or some other elaborate dish. Some of us were able to do this because they risked their lives so that we could. It dawned on us the significance of these COVID fighters. An international epidemic forced us to reflect on what is actually significant in life.

So far, at least 6 million people's lives have been cut short by the Covid-19 pandemic. Death rates among the elderly are very high, therefore experts believe the true death toll might be two or even four times higher. Many more millions will have to deal with "long Covid," or handicap because of their illness. For months at a time, nearly two billion children and young adults had their schooling halted.

Education was the hardest hit by the pandemic. Millions of young girls around the world, especially children of color stopped going to school and cannot afford to return.

As a result of the pandemic, many young people were forced into undesirable roles such as marriage, fatherhood, and/or work. The reasons were not farfetched as nearly half a billion people fell into poverty or lost their means of earning an income due to the pandemic. Additionally, billions more are dealing with the effects of the economic slowdown it caused.

As the pandemic enters its fourth year, the disparities that have marked its first two years become even more ingrained. Huge inequalities in vaccine access persist around the world, even 15 months after the World Health Organization authorized the first Covid-19 vaccine in an emergency situation. Even though some people are getting second or even third doses of vaccines, over 85% of those who live in low-income countries have yet to receive even the first.

We are still in the midst of a widespread Covid-19 epidemic. At the start of the third year of the epidemic, New Zealand, South Korea, Hong Kong, and Vietnam are all experiencing their largest documented waves of infections since the pandemic was proclaimed in March 2020. It's a question that's being asked around the world by a lot of people: What could have been done differently?

Human Rights Watch's research during the past two years of the pandemic sheds light on both governments' failures to meet human rights duties and opportunistic attempts to use the outbreak as a pretext to extend authorities, crush opponents, and repress dissent. We show how things may have turned out differently if human rights had been prioritized in more policy responses, which is the focus of our investigation. It also suggests a fairer path forward.

In this chapter, we will look back on the pandemic and the lessons it taught us.

• THE VALUE of Independence

THE PANDEMIC MADE us realize the need of having a plan for a lockdown and being responsible for our own safety at home. We recognized our innate need for the care of our parents, caregivers, and other loved ones. We realized how much we relied on our domestic help and took them for granted when they did things like cleaning, laundry, and dishes for us. The coronavirus brought the globe to its knees, but it also taught us an important lesson about the power of compassion. After being cooped up for over a year, we've become more self-reliant and resourceful than ever before.

. . .

● ESSENTIAL MEDICAL Supplies should be Easily Accessible, Cheap, & Available to Anyone Who Needs Them.

HEALTH, lives, and livelihoods are still at risk due to unequal access to cost-effective Covid-19 vaccinations. In order to increase and diversify worldwide manufacturing of Covid-19 vaccines, it is necessary for pharmaceutical companies and the governments that sponsor them to agree to share information and technology. So, while approximately 11 billion doses of Covid-19 vaccine have been provided worldwide as we enter year three, in low and middle income nations millions of doctors, frontline workers, and individuals at high risk of severe disease and death are still waiting for their first shot. As safe and effective medications became available on the market, the same dynamics we've seen with vaccination access were repeated, despite some pledges allowing for the more diverse manufacture of antiviral tablets. Instead than being an inevitable byproduct of market shortages, the failure of governments to meet their human rights commitments to share the benefits of scientific research to defend the rights to life, health, and a decent standard of living is the root cause of this inequality.

• THERE IS NO MORE Important Entity than Family

ANOTHER INSIGHT that has come to us in the past year and a half is the significance of our family. During this terrifying time, many people chose to stay alone and talk about what it was like to be so far from home and constantly fear for their own and their loved ones' safety. Those who were at home described some of their most memorable family bonding experiences. Some worked on improving their cooking abilities, some did duties around the house, and yet others spent their time playing board games. It was agreed upon that the experience of the epidemic brought people closer together, reducing the gulf between them and their loved ones.

• SMALL PLEASURES Can Bring Big Smiles

. . .

THEY HAD no idea that their lives would suddenly change for the worst, and they would be grounded for what felt like an eternity. We were too preoccupied with the big picture to notice the small victories along the way. Those who had lost their sense of smell or taste owing to COVID-19 described how much they enjoyed home-cooked meals once they regained their senses. How working out hard had never felt better, how playing games together as a family had strengthened their bonds. These are the minutiae that we took for granted a year ago but now eagerly anticipate each day. Time has come for us to value them and our possessions.

• CARE for Your Mental Health As It Matters

AS A SPECIES, humans need the company of others in order to feel secure and cared for emotionally. The number of people with mental health issues in India is estimated to be around 30 million. However, only a small percentage really gets help. In light of the widespread spread of the coronavirus in India, we were forced to go into quarantine. Physical contact is reduced as a result of increased isolation, social withdrawal, telecommuting, and online education. Despite the urgency of the situation, it's crucial to keep in touch with loved ones. Increasing your serotonin levels and giving you more energy, a good diet and regular exercise can do wonders. One method to protect our mental health is to avoid exposure to misleading information. Sharing positive stories and keeping the spirits up can help us all get through tough times.

• A LITTLE Act of Kindness Can Mean the World

WHEN DISCUSSING the importance of mental wellness, it is important to remember that our words and deeds can have a significant impact on the emotional well-being of those around us. It's best to be nice to everyone because we can never know what they're going through. Complimenting someone, assisting the elderly, bringing groceries to a sick neighbor, or simply providing reliable information online can all make a difference in someone's life. We can all feel at peace if we do what we can to spread happiness at this time of unrest caused by the pandemic. Feelings of anxiety and stress can be reduced by practicing gratitude and counting one's blessings.

● TECHNOLOGY BECOME **Our Best Friend**

OF COURSE, the world has long been going digital. However, before the pandemic, it was common practice for most senior citizens in the United States to go to the grocery store, put on shoes, get their blood pressure checked, and then watch the latest blockbuster in theaters.

It is possible that the digital answer will become many Americans' first choice for dealing with life's duties, and this will be the most far-reaching social effect of the pandemic. Despite our continued clinging to certain "IRL" (in real life) encounters, it is becoming clear that user-friendly, cutting-edge virtual tools are the new norm.

If nothing else, COVID has shown us how robust and adaptive humans are as a society when forced to change. In order to keep living and communicating with our loved ones during the epidemic, we've been forced to master new technologies that, in many circumstances, have been the only safe means to continue to do so.

The rise of technology was about more than just Skype and Netflix. The profits of well-known applications that arrange for the delivery of meals more than doubled in 2017. Services like weddings and funerals were held virtually (sure, we will return to in-person gatherings, but likely with cameras and live feeds to include distant attendees). PayPal indicated that its fastest-growing user category was persons over the age of 50, and Chase said that around half of its new online users were in this age range. More and more regular medical checkups are being performed via webcam, thanks to telehealth, and insurance companies are beginning to pay for these visits. This method soon became the only option to operate at scale in today's environment, for both themselves and their patients. Even after COVID is no longer active, telemedicine will prove to be a superior and more efficient option for many patients.

10

WHERE DO WE GO FROM HERE?

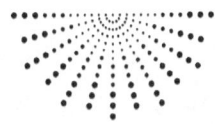

here Are We Right Now?

Who might have anticipated that a worldwide pandemic and an economic catastrophe would be the catalysts for evaluating our place in the universe?

The global spread of COVID-19 has been like a tsunami. It has shown no tolerance, spreading the virus irrespective of faith, class, or money, disregarding state identities, demanding attention, and pushing over any efforts at maintaining 'business as usual'.

The terrible side of human greed was on full display as people stocked up on perceived necessities at the expense of others, disregarded calls for them to stay inside, and refused to maintain any sort of emotional distance.

Nevertheless, it has also shown the resilience of our community, as thousands of people have offered their time to help, and waves of applause have traveled throughout the country to honor our most vital employees. These are true heroes, risking their lives every day to provide essential services, combat the virus, and care for the sick and the weak.

As a result of equipment and facility shortages, we have seen companies shift their attention away from competition and toward product and service innovation.

More time is being spent within households. People now have more time on their hands, and with that comes a rediscovered appreciation for the outdoors and natural phenomena. People are now walking to their destinations when they would previously have taken vehicles or buses. A lot of folks we know are doing their farming, baking their bread, and supporting their local farmers' markets.

Notwithstanding the COVID-19 crisis's numerous devastating consequences in the form of disease and mortality, it is precisely what we required to galvanize us, to draw us together as one global community, to see much more of the goals we are cooperatively in a position to accomplish and to bring into focus what is necessary internationally to protect our future on this planet.

The economic cycle has been broken or at least temporarily thrown off. It's too late to go back to our old ways of doing things, but perhaps it's for the better that things are different now. A new normal has emerged as people look for explanations for the changes that have taken place.

From the beginning of the COVID-19 epidemic for over 3 years ago, a lot has happened. Telemedicine, virtual conferences, and online residency/fellowship interviews are just some examples of how the requirement for social separation has spurred the digitization of healthcare delivery and medical education.

Because of research and development in the field of mRNA technology, safe and effective vaccines are now readily available. As the number of people who recover from an acute infection increases, so does the number of people who require medical care for chronic infection. Furthermore, numerous misinformation campaigns have been fueled by social media platforms, which have had an impact on control and preventative efforts.

What is currently a burden for us may soon become a boon. The expression "necessity is the mother of invention" rings true.

As the traditional methods of doing things crumble under the weight of the current global crisis, we are forced to take notice of the emerging new ones.

Virtual work has expanded at an unprecedented rate due to the prevalence of mandatory isolation policies. Many traditionally in-person corporate tasks, such as meetings, coaching, briefings, presentations, and conferences, have moved online. The internet has become increasingly important in our daily lives, whether for work, school, or just plain fun.

Spending less money and potentially helping the environment are two benefits of working virtually.

The normal chaos of the day has subsided, allowing us to reflect. The good and the bad can both be considered in light of our past experiences. Together, we can begin to envision a future in which our altered actions put us in better harmony with the natural world.

Newly established "no-fly zones" have resulted in cleaner air, spurring discussions about the possibility of reducing expensive business trips while simultaneously lowering atmospheric pollution. Substantial cuts on emissions from gasoline and diesel automobiles have led to cleaner air in urban centers. As a result of the lockdown, even the canals of Venice are cleaner than they have been in years, and fish have begun to return.

Greenhouse gas emissions reduce dramatically as industrial production declines. According to data collected by the Finnish Centre for Research on Energy and Clean Air in the four weeks beginning in late January, Chinese carbon dioxide emissions decreased by 25% when compared to the corresponding period in 2017.

What about the food that we consume? One theory puts the responsibility for the spread of COVID-19 on zoonosis, the spread of disease from animals to humans. Even though scientists have only just begun to piece together what led to the outbreak of the virus, they have already linked intense, industrial-scale farming to the creation of hybrid strains of meat.

It's been debated whether or not it's morally acceptable for us to buy and eat food that's been produced in other countries and shipped here. Is it okay to eat fruit when it's not in season or to consume fish from overfished waters?

After a string of extreme weather events, including floods, hurricanes, fires, droughts, and ice melts, COVID-19 finally made landfall. The current coronavirus pandemic is not the only hazard to our global society; climate change and the continued loss of biodiversity pose equally serious risks. I would guess there are more.

There has been a heightened awareness among corporations, governments, and communities on the importance of addressing various risks to humanity. As they have more knowledge and expertise, they should take charge. Many people are talking about how the climate issue can benefit from the new paradigm that has emerged as a result of the social crisis.

There is a new transformation agenda that is gathering support and posing persistent questions.

It's getting dangerously close to the breaking point for some businesses. They find out that their business models can't last. They are vulnerable because they rely on an inefficient, isolated service activity that can be readily uncovered and disrupted. All of this offers an ideal environment for commercially driven, long-term innovations that drastically alter how companies operate and how their customers behave.

Leaders who are open to new ideas and methods of operation are urgently needed around the globe. Leadership that frees up genius and uses it to propel transformation, repair the environment, and create new norms is essential.

Now the pieces begin to fit together. The big image is gradually taking shape before our eyes. We're learning a lot from our time spent against COVID-19. It is our responsibility to use these insights to address the climate problem, which is likely the most severe threat humanity has ever faced. As we cope with COVID-19, we may learn lessons that influence how we act in the future.

. . .

So, WHERE ARE WE RIGHT NOW?

ONLY AFTER THE Covid epidemic can we make any kind of long-term predictions on each of the forecasts. Some are more optimistic than others. Despite this unparalleled setback, nearly everyone believes that civilization can and will eventually bounce back.

Our homes, as well as our values, lifestyles, and habits, will all evolve as a result. Seven possible future developments are forecasted below.

The purpose of tall structures is to house a large number of people in a well-organized and manageable manner. There were zero regard for people's health and cleanliness. In the event of a pandemic, residents of high-rise buildings should take extra precautions to limit their exposure to the virus by avoiding close contact with the elevators, buttons, door handles, surfaces, and, most importantly, their neighbors.

We will all long for a home more than ever after being isolated from one another for so long on different floors above ground, often without a balcony or terrace. Despite its modest size, it should have a patio or courtyard where you can enjoy your morning coffee.

The primary purpose of the home throughout history has been to provide a haven. At first, it was a haven from the elements and predators. In that era, formidable stone fortifications were constructed to keep out hostile forces. People in the modern era require a home that can successfully isolate them from the outside world.

The house is now more of a sanctuary from illness than from the monotony of daily life or the craziness of the city. When more people choose to live in suburban or rural areas, urbanization slows down.

The structures of the future will be strong and self-sufficient, providing for their own water and heating needs. The use of geothermal wells is becoming increasingly common. Besides providing water, they can also contribute to a household's energy needs by warming the air inside.

Stoves, fireplaces, solid fuel boilers, fuel generators, and solar panels will all be available as backup heating options. Mini-stations that can run independently and produce renewable energy are on the horizon. The plan is to become self-sufficient in the event of a total blackout, reducing vulnerability as much as possible.

Now, only a few groups of people and businesses, including those in the maritime industry, the construction industry, and the armed forces, have access to satellite internet due to its prohibitive cost and inconvenient availability. As advances speed up civilian applications, we can look forward to lightning-fast internet speeds.

Even before the epidemic hit, OneWeb and SpaceX had planned to use this technology to blanket the entire planet. Although just 40 of OneWeb's 648 satellites have been launched into Earth's orbit so far, SpaceX's Starlink project anticipates the launch of 12,000 satellites into low orbit by the middle of the 2020s.

VERY FASCINATING, **wouldn't you say?**

MOST PEOPLE HAVE to stay at home and work throughout the quarantine period. Some people will be eager to see their coworkers and get their caffeine fix the moment the quarantine is lifted. But, other people just can't imagine going back to work.

There will be a heightened focus on optimal home office layout. The traditional setup of a home office—a desk in the corner of the living room or hidden away under the stairs with a lamp and a chair that looks like they belong in a parody of an office—will soon become obsolete. This new space is going to be entirely isolated from the rest of the house and will have big windows, blackout curtains, and plush furnishings. It will be soundproofed and fitted with the latest technology.

As a result, government agencies will exert greater effort in their pursuit of our patronage. Eventually, the features enjoyed by the most innovative businesses today will be standard fare.

Time has shown, however, that many of the most troubling aspects of this issue are not novel. Existing economic inequalities may account for the striking discrepancies in COVID-19 infections and outcomes. Due to the all-too-familiar market's inability to properly value what counts, "important workers" often receive shockingly low compensation despite contributing greatly to society.

With populism on the rise and trust in specialists at an all-time low, it was to be expected that people would enthusiastically embrace false information about the virus. With the current glorification of "my country first" global politics, the lack of a fully coordinated international response should hardly have been unexpected.

In this sense, the crisis is a revelation because it highlights the many preexisting inequalities and frailties in our social order. Even if previous audiences failed to recognize these flaws, they should be obvious now.

After the dust settles from COVID-19, how would the world look like? There will be a lot of difficulties in the coming decade, but many of them will be magnified forms of issues we have now. Upon emerging from this crisis, if we decide to take action to fix these challenges and bring about profound change, the world will look very different this time.

The narrative of this book has taken us from the beginning of vaccine use to the present, covering the history of vaccination injuries, delving deeply into the controversial lockdown, vaccine, and big Pharma partnership, searching for a natural solution and pondering the pandemic as a whole. If you've been following along since the beginning, you know there's some debate around COVID-19 and LOCKDOWN in general, and you know that things aren't going back to normal anytime soon. The effects of the pandemic are hastening or challenging several ongoing developments in the global economy.

- Challenges we have to confront as a global system; important challenges.
- Challenges that require our immediate attention.
- Challenges, if solved immediately, could help us live in harmony with nature.

IT'S past time to do something about it and make some changes.

Will you be part of this? Where will you be? In this uncharted territory where we find ourselves right now?

. . .

Conclusion

Why the pandemic was widely disapproved by many people?

Aspects of the lockdown that weren't right

- **Vague explanation of what was really happening**

This served as a serious problem in managing the virus. A lot of people lacked past basic knowledge of the pandemic during the lockdown phase. Many conspiracy theories started popping up, as some blamed China, the elites, and in some parts of Africa, it was believed to be retaliation from the deities for the diminishing belief of their followers.

As a result, fear began to creep in, causing a large percent of deaths during that period. There was even a record of highly salted water being a cure for the virus, and as expected, it did no more than damage the internal organs of its consumers. The public health systems didn't do well in the initial explanation of the problem and its solutions or possible preventive measures, hence leaving the people misguided like a snake without a head.

POSSIBLE ALTERNATIVES TO MASS LOCKDOWN AND QUARANTINE PROCEDURES IN THE INCIDENT OF ANOTHER COVID-19 WAVE

A WELL DREADED event is a new wave of COVID-19 cases, but the future is and will remain unpredictable. Therefore, it is important to explore alternatives to the mass lockdown and quarantine procedures used during the first phase of the pandemic, which were highly disruptive and resulted in significant economic and social impacts during the earlier wave. It is certain that the masses would not comply with such a trample on their fundamental human rights again, so instead of a stay-at-home initiative, authorities may consider implementing less one-sided measures that can be easily adhered to by citizens, and that facilitate a healing process without difficult scars.

The first COVID-19 wave could be defined as the perfect preparation phase for governments, citizens, and health sectors all across the globe. With its unexpected arrival, and hastened widespread, it was an accurate test on how quickly we can respond to such stimuli.

Till this moment, not even an 80% come-back from the crippling disadvantages of that period can be bragged about by any nation of the world. So, if the proper lessons have actually been learnt, why take the world through such a route when there are multiple alternatives?

Some of the possible steps that would control the virus, and at the same time maintain the usual lives of individuals.

STRICT SOCIAL DISTANCING INSTEAD of a total lockdown

WE WILL KICK off with strict social distancing, which can be more productive than a total lockdown. Quoting the Deputy Editor of The Economist, Edward Carr, "the lockdown was just a really intense form of social distancing." And not only was it intense, it punctuated all normal activities. Such a policy would involve limiting the number of individuals that can visit public places, rotating work and class hours, and imposing customer limits per hour in stores, among other methods. It was a notable feature of the earlier phases of China's return from the first phase of the pandemic. These measures would reduce the likelihood of contact between individuals, while enabling normal activities to continue.

TESTING AND TRACING

LOOKING at the social distancing technique, a lot of concerns will surely be raised due to the possibility of high infection rate. That is when you employ the test and trace mechanism, which involves tracking down infected individuals through contact tracing.

This can be achieved through mobile apps, similar to those developed by Germany, Ireland, and the USA during the earlier wave.

Such an innovation would be able to keep track of contacts made by an individual, so once a positive case is confirmed, all contacts made by such a person would be brought in for testing and isolation, to ensure that the virus doesn't spread further. This approach would enable authorities to isolate only confirmed cases, rather than imposing quarantine on everybody. It will also prevent those who have come in contact with the virus to start early treatments, so as to hasten their recovery.

Vaccination

Proper vaccination would also be crucial in controlling the virus. The preventive COVID-19 vaccine would be administered to individuals who are not infected or come across the virus at any point, while patients who have tested positive undergo treatment. It is also important to have the people's trust, so it will be sensible to set up public vaccination units in common places like places of religious worships, workplaces, schools, universities, and other common places, as it has been proven that a large percentage of the world's population face Nosocomephobia, which is the fear of visiting hospitals and health centers for treatment. This is as a result of the uncertainty that is conjoined with going into a hospital.

EDUCATION AND ENLIGHTENMENT

IT IS a major failure during the first phase, as most people didn't know past the basics of what was really going on. When there is no information, there's no power, hence being the cause of the defiance and breaching of COVID-19 policies.

At the advent of another phase, it would be important for authorities to provide clear and accurate information to the public about the virus, its preventive measures, and the vaccines. Failure to provide such information during the earlier wave led to widespread fear, confusion, and misinformation, which contributed to a large percentage of the mortality recorded.

In light of this, world organizations like the UN, EU, and other humanitarian and financial bodies should work hand in hand to manage such a situation, as they lacked show of cooperation during the first phase.

11

CONCLUSION

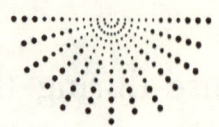

*A*s I conclude this book by saying, I am filled with a sense of urgency and hope. The challenges we face as a species and a planet are daunting, but they are not insurmountable. We have the power, the knowledge, and the resources to create a better world, but we need to act now.

We need to wake up and see what is happening to us. Humanity and the world are in trouble. If we don't wake up and take action, we are at risk of losing our freedom and literally the life expectancy of most vaxxed are only 3-5 years if not addressed! We need to acknowledge the interconnectedness of our problems and address them with urgency and collective effort. We need to transcend our differences and work together for the common good.

We need to see beyond the illusions that separate us. We need to stop dividing ourselves through race, religion, political views, gender, vaxxed or not-vaxxed. We need to realize that we are all connected and that our fates are intertwined. We need to embrace a sense of empathy and compassion for all living beings and the planet we share.

Love is a powerful force that can help us overcome the challenges we face. Love can inspire us to take action, to make sacrifices, and to work towards a better future. Love can help us overcome fear, anger, and hatred, and it can create a sense of unity and solidarity. Love can win over evil, and it can heal the wounds of the world.

But love alone is not enough. We also need to take concrete actions to address the problems we face. We need to not give our trust and powers over to evil forces like the WHO and Gates. We need to shift our focus from consumption to conservation, from competition to cooperation, and from exploitation to stewardship. We need to invest in renewable energy, green infrastructure, and sustainable agriculture. We need to reform our economic and political systems to make them more just and equitable. We need to educate ourselves and our children about the challenges we face and the solutions that are available.

We also need to acknowledge the power of natural healing. Our bodies and minds have an incredible capacity to heal themselves, and there are many natural remedies and practices that can help us achieve optimal health and well-being. We need to shift our focus from reactive medicine to proactive medicine, and we need to embrace a holistic approach.

We are powerful and capable of doing anything, including healing and turning this world into a place of love and peace. You can make a difference. We can make a difference! We need to act now, and we need to act together. The future of humanity and the planet depends on our actions today.

In conclusion, let us wake up and see what is happening to us. Let us acknowledge the challenges we face and take action with urgency and collective effort. Let us transcend our differences and embrace our interconnectedness. Let us harness the power of love, natural healing, and collective action to create a better world. We have the power to create a future that is just, sustainable, and full of hope. Let us seize this opportunity and make it a reality.

You deserve to live a life free of suffering and pain. You deserve to be free of all disease and illness. It is yours for the taking; all you have to do is make that choice.

Thank you for your courage and open-mindedness in reading this book. You are now on the right path to gaining more knowledge, insight, and wisdom toward your healing. I truly wish you nothing but perfect health so that you can enjoy your life full of happiness.

Next Steps:

1.) If you enjoyed this book, please leave an honest review on Amazon.

2.) If you send me a screenshot of your review then you will receive a 30-minute complementary consultation valued at $125.

3.) If you want to learn how we can help you attain that self-healing power, reach out to us through email: **Skye8Angelou@gmail.com**

12

ABOUT THE AUTHOR

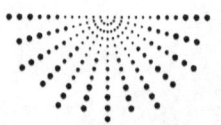

$\mathcal{S}$kye Angelou is a believer in all things possible. Skye also believes that self-healing can be attained under the right conditions. Over 3 decades, the focus has been on restoring, reviving, and rebuilding what was lost to sickness and conventional medicine.

Skye is not your average healer, but a clever, fearless, and spiritual being ready to help facilitate healing for the next person. And could it be you?

Skye Angelou is a beautiful soul that aligns with the universe and happiness from being able to re-direct people's disbelief about self-healing to a place where they experience 100% personal health renewal of mind, body, and soul. There is no reason why you cannot enjoy the same level of health as those helped thus far.

Healing is your right. You deserve the right to a healthier, livelier and more fulfilling quality of life. CLAIM IT NOW! **Connect with Skye today. Skye8Angelou@gmail.com**